TALES FROM KENTUCKY
ONE-ROOM SCHOOL TEACHERS

TALES FROM

KENTUCKY ONE-ROOM SCHOOL TEACHERS

William Lynwood Montell

THE UNIVERSITY PRESS OF KENTUCKY

Scholarly publisher for the Commonwealth,
serving Bellarmine University, Berea College, Centre
College of Kentucky, Eastern Kentucky University,
The Filson Historical Society, Georgetown College,
Kentucky Historical Society, Kentucky State University,
Morehead State University, Murray State University,
Northern Kentucky University, Transylvania University,
University of Kentucky, University of Louisville,
and Western Kentucky University.
All rights reserved.

Editorial and Sales Offices: The University Press of Kentucky
663 South Limestone Street, Lexington, Kentucky 40508-4008
www.kentuckypress.com

15 14 13 12 11   5 4 3 2 1

Library of Congress Cataloging-in-Publication Data
Montell, William Lynwood, 1931–
  Tales from Kentucky one-room school teachers / William Lynwood
Montell.
        p.   cm.
  Includes bibliographical references and index.
  ISBN 978-0-8131-2979-2 (hardcover : alk. paper) —
  ISBN 978-0-8131-2980-8 (ebook)
  1. Education—Kentucky—History. 2. Teaching—Kentucy—History.
3. Teachers—Kentucky—History. 4. Tales—Kentucky. 5. Kentucky—Social
life and customs. I. Title.
  LA292.M66 2011
  372.12'509769—dc22
                              2010044909

This book is printed on acid-free recycled paper meeting
the requirements of the American National Standard
for Permanence in Paper for Printed Library Materials.

Manufactured in the United States of America.

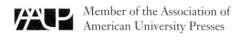

Member of the Association of
American University Presses

CONTENTS

Introduction

When I came back to the schoolroom from the outhouse one morning, teacher Jerry Bowman beckoned me over to him and whispered, "Lynwood, button up your britches—you forgot to do it!"

The era of the Kentucky one-room schoolhouse represents a facet of the educational profession that no longer exists. Kentucky lost an abundant amount of its social, cultural, and educational heritage when its one-room schools were closed. I conceived this collection to gather valuable oral history of this unique period from former one-room school teachers across the Commonwealth, knowing that they could share fabulous stories and historical information that would otherwise be lost to us when those who can tell these stories have left us for good.

My purpose in recording the memories of these old-time teachers, most of whom were in their nineties or older, was to help preserve the legacy and contributions of this particular sector of Kentucky history. This book provides descriptive accounts of what the one-room school era was like for teachers, students, and the wider community, encompassing school infrastructure, school events both typical and unusual, teacher-student relationships, and other factors relative to the culture of an educational system that began in pioneer times and ended during the 1950s to the 1970s, primarily in the 1960s.

Historical information passed along verbally is a significant and valuable source of data that complements formal historiographical sources. Combining the two sectors of knowledge forms a fuller historical record: formal historiography provides objective interpretation based on information on file, and oral history offers an insightful personal touch. Oral history methodology helps to achieve invaluable perspectives on local culture.

It should be noted that none of the oral accounts in this book are universal, a term used by folklorists in reference to verbal stories that are told statewide, nationwide, or even worldwide in some instances. Folklorists study and reproduce universal legends in some instances, but they are primarily interested in meaningful individual stories that describe a local culture at a particular point in time. This is true of oral history, "which is both the method by which verbal information about the past and/or present is collected and recorded, and the body of knowledge that exists only in people's memories, which will be lost when they and other members of their generation have died. . . . Orally communicated history can supplement written records by filling in the gaps in formal documents or providing an insider's perspective on momentous events."[1] Many of the teachers' stories herein do reveal these inside perspectives and viewpoints that make oral history projects such vital scholarship.

At the heart of this scholarship is an intensely personal human process: this book's evocation of the wonderful heritage of Kentucky's one-room school era is thanks to the many former teachers who shared their stories—by turns laugh-out-loud funny, heartwarming, poignant, sad, and even frightening—and were thrilled for the opportunity to do so. Often they spoke with tears in their eyes.

To locate my interview subjects, I contacted Brenda Meredith, editor of the quarterly publication *KRTA (Kentucky Retired Teachers Association) News* and explained my intended project. She asked me to write an explanatory letter for inclusion in the December 2008 issue. I very quickly began getting responses from former one-room school teachers in several counties across the state. After initial contact with prospective storytellers by telephone or e-mail, I wrote a letter to them, including a set of questions intended to suggest story and viewpoint categories for them to ponder. Then, depending on the interviewees' preference, I either drove to their residence to tape-record their memories or they sent me tape-recorded or written accounts, the latter by e-mail or regular mail. All three of the suggested methods were employed, almost evenly. Meeting face-to-face with these former one-room school teachers to interview them was truly an honor as well as a fascinating venture. For their part, the teachers were friendly and excited to be participating in my project. I was also in contact with many others whom I never met personally but talked with on the telephone or communicated with via e-mail. (I am particularly thankful that I had the opportunity to interview Mamie Wright, one of my own three one-room school teachers, just two weeks before her death.)

Union College, located in Barbourville, Knox County, was also of monumental service in obtaining names, telephone numbers, e-mail addresses, and regular mail addresses of former one-room school teachers in Knox and other counties. Once the needed information was obtained, very helpful Union College staff members invited all the teachers and me to be present at a two-day storytelling/recording event.

After inputting all the stories onto my computer disk, I mailed each storyteller a copy of his or her story. In my cover letter I wrote, "I have transcribed the stories and viewpoints you told [sent] and have included a copy of each one for you to read and make needed editorial changes. Write any needed corrections, additions, deletions, etc., on the pages, them send me all pages on which you make changes. I will then place the changes on my computer disk." All of these cooperative former teachers did indeed return editorial changes as necessary. Thus the stories in this book appear exactly as their tellers intended them.

I regret that more Kentucky counties are not represented in this book, despite my best efforts. Counties represented in this book are Adair, Barren, Bell, Boone, Breckinridge, Butler, Caldwell, Carter, Clinton, Crittenden, Cumberland, Daviess, Edmonson, Estill, Floyd, Grayson, Green, Greenup, Hardin, Henry, Johnson, Knox, Laurel, Letcher, Logan, Lyon, Magoffin, Marion, Marshall, Metcalfe, Monroe, Morgan, Muhlenberg, Ohio, Pike, Rockcastle, Russell, Spencer, Taylor, Trimble, Warren, Washington, and Wayne. Other counties are not included because I was unable to locate there any living former one-room school teachers, the teachers declined my invitation, or people simply did not have adequate memories of their early teaching years.

Story categories included in the book are "Initial Teaching Years," "Teaching Methods and Philosophy," "Bad Boys and Girls," "Vignettes of One-Room Schoolhouse Life," "Disciplining Students," "Daily Activities," "Outhouses," "Getting to and from School," "Teacher and Community Relations," "Students with Special Needs," "Before and After Consolidation," and "Home Life of Students." (The teachers' biographies included at the end of the book, provided by the subjects, are themselves stories.) Each story grouping is described in the introduction to its chapter. Of course, the bulk of these stories are relevant to the personal involvement of the teacher who tells the story, even if the tale relates to student behavior, and thus the storytellers themselves are the central focus, making these personal memories truly historic treasures. At the same time, through the alchemy of storytelling, a panorama of the period emerges.

In 1872 the Kentucky State Legislature formally mandated its nine "Rules for Teachers":

1. Teachers each day will fill lamps, trim the wicks and clean chimneys.
2. Each morning teacher will bring a bucket of water and a scuttle of coal for the day's session.
3. Make your pens carefully. You may whittle nibs to the individual taste of the pupils.
4. Men teachers may take one evening each week for courting purposes, or two evenings a week if they attend church regularly.
5. After ten hours in school, the teachers may spend the remaining time reading the Bible or any other good books.
6. Women teachers who marry or engage in unseemly conduct will be dismissed.
7. Every teacher should lay aside from each pay a goodly sum of his earnings for his benefit during his declining years so that he will not become a burden on society.
8. Any teacher who smokes, uses liquor in any form, frequents pool or public halls, or gets shaved in a barber shop will give good cause to suspect his worth, intention, integrity and honesty.
9. The teacher who performs his labor faithfully and without fault for five years will be given an increase of twenty-five cents per week for his pay, providing the Board of Education approves.[2]

In reference to Crittenden County and likely other counties across the state, "Few of the teachers made teaching their regular business. A few were ministers who taught during the week and were educated; others were rough and not very gentlemanly. Ladies were seldom employed as teachers because they were not supposed to know enough."[3]

A word about the physical infrastructure of one-room school buildings might be helpful here in enabling the reader to visualize the scenes of the stories in this book. Most such buildings constructed in the 1800s were small, typically built by using logs subsequently covered with board planks. The heating facility was a fireplace built with large rocks. A doorway and one or two windows were opened by cutting out adequate spaces in the log walls. Seats for the students were made of wooden slabs supported by pins or logs at each end and had no backs.[4]

Very few of the original log school buildings are still standing, though those that remain are protected as historical landmarks. Likewise, very few of the sawed wooden plank/frame buildings that were constructed, typically beginning in the mid- to late 1880s, are still standing. Those that remain are either being preserved as school museums or are, sadly, rotting away.

In the rural districts where these one-room school buildings once stood, they played a significant role in the community, serving not only as schools but as social centers. The local school building was variously used as a venue for political speeches, as a movie theater, and as a gathering place for all kinds of social get-togethers. In many communities, church services, including annual revival services, were sometimes held in these schools.[5]

The present book is not intended to serve only historians or educators, although I hope that scholars will use it as required reading for students in the field of education. Rather, I envision a general audience. It is hoped that reading these stories will foster for those who attended a one-room school fond—perhaps even bittersweet—memories of their own. For those who know very little about the one-room school era, but who would like to better understand what educational conditions were like in the past, the stories will provide insightful knowledge of Kentucky's educational history. The stories and thoughts expressed by these former teachers are an important aspect of Kentucky's cultural legacy.

I truly have a deep appreciation for the men and women who took the time to share their memories for inclusion in this book. Teachers made and continue to make incalculable contributions to our society. Some former students of Kentucky's one-room schools still hold reunions to honor their schoolteachers. In a different but no less heartfelt way, this book is intended as a similar tribute.

Notes

1. William Lynwood Montell, *Tales from Tennessee Lawyers* (Lexington: University Press of Kentucky, 2005), 5.

2. Alma Jean Hocker, comp., *Butler County Schools*, vol. 1, *In the Early Days* (Morgantown, Ky.: Embrys of Morgantown, 1996), 6.

3. Crittenden County Historical Society, *History of Crittenden County Schools, 1842–1987* (Utica, Ky.: McDowell, 1987), 2.

4. Ibid.

5. Hocker, *Butler County Schools*, 6.

Further Reading

Hartford, Ellis. *The Little White School House.* Lexington: University Press of Kentucky, 1977.

Smith, Daniel T. "Appalachia's Last One-Room School: A Case Study." Ph.D. diss., University of Kentucky, 1988.

Williams, Cratis. *I Became a Teacher: A Memoir of One-Room School Life in Eastern Kentucky.* Ashland, Ky.: Jesse Stuart Foundation, 1995.

Chapter 1

Initial Teaching Years

In this section teachers share memories of their teaching careers, encompassing stories describing the very first day of class presided over by a nervous young teacher—perhaps only a year or two older than some of her students—to retrospective thoughts on a career lasting decades. In between are portraits of individual rural schools, an overview of what teaching in Kentucky's one-room schools was truly like for those in the front lines. Teachers' salaries, their daily duties, the conditions they encountered in the schools, their hardships and rewards—and, most importantly, their students—are all depicted here.

Late Nineteenth-Century Teaching

I secured a school at Flenersville, Butler County. Mr. John Satterfield was Trustee of this district. I had a very large school, several pupils older than myself. I was only in my 17th year. School age was from 6 to 20 yr. One man 25 years old applied for entrance and through the advice given by the Trustee he became one of my students, and a very good one he was. He entered this school only a 3rd grader but became so interested he continued in his home school 2 or 3 years longer, then went to Morgantown for 2 or 3 years, and when I left Butler County he was expecting to teach the next fall. I heard later he taught for several years in Butler and Ohio counties. He bore the very common name of Bill Bratcher. I think I labored as hard with this school of 50 boys and girls as I ever did in any school I ever tried to teach. Only a boy 17 years old and with only a Second Class Third Grade Certificate, I apparently gave satisfaction as the whole school both pupils and patrons insisted I should offer my services again. I began the first Monday in August 1878 and closed out the 5th month Friday before Christmas. Next summer I drew ninety-four dollars from the state for my services rendered. . . .

In January of 1876 I entered [taught] a three months school taught by Kiah McKinney. I taught the next year at Shallow Ford (Sycamore) in Butler County. Wylie Daugherty was Trustee. This was a new house and I was its first teacher. The house was built on a hillside, one door only entering from the lower end of the house and required, as I recollect, four steps to reach. The upper end was on ground. There was a snug fireplace here, and a small window on each side. This was claimed by these people to be the warmest, best lighted, and best ventilated school house in the county north of the Green River. I know it was plenty warm in summer, being located in an old thrown out field with no trees located near it, and would roast you in winter if you could get enough wood up those steps to make a fire. About 55 of us smothered and roasted by turns according to the seasons. I received one hundred twenty dollars for trying to teach this school, and made some very warm friends here. Three of the boys who attended this school afterward went beyond the eighth grade. One was Owen Daugherty who taught several years, then studied pharmacy and ran a drug store in Caneyville. The others were Steve and Mac Cook, each of whom taught. Mac, the last I heard of him, was county judge of Ohio County, and Steve in the mercantile business, also in Ohio County. . . .

In the winter of 1878 I came to Warren County to attend school at Plum Springs. James W. Simmons was the teacher. I boarded with John A. Bryant at what is now known as the McDaniel place. There were about 25 young men and women in attendance here. I was again examined this year in Brownsville, making a Second Class, Second Grade Certificate, and taught this year at Hawk's schoolhouse near Glenmore. A Mr. Meredith was School Commissioner of Edmonson County at this time. I boarded with Mr. Simmons during this year which was out Jan. 17th, 1879. I walked home the next day, a distance of about 35 miles. I had a large school at this place but only one pupil who ever passed beyond 8th grade, who was Rochester Watt, now teaching in Georgia. The teachers didn't draw their pay for this year until July of the next year, so I had to make a trip to Brownsville by way of Brooklyn, Lumbustown, Reedyville, across Bear Creek, where I also crossed the line from Butler County into Edmonson County and went on into Brownsville. This stretch of 12 or 15 miles was sparsely settled and reported to be rather dangerous. I had to make the trip by myself and thought I needed some sort of way to protect myself if I encountered [danger] and [had] need of protection. I mentioned my fears to two boys or young men who readily offered to loan me their pistols. I readily accepted, thinking if one was any protection, two would be twice as much, so I went on my way over this supposedly dangerous road feeling somewhat safe. I arrived in Brownsville about 4 o'clock in the evening without anything dangerous or unusual happening on the road. But when I arrived here I found the Superintendent had gone home, which was at Bee Springs, about 9 miles away. Well, I had to follow him, which was over the lonesomest road I ever traveled. I passed only two houses of the entire way. I found him to be a very clever and pleasant old gentleman. It being late and I being tired, I only too gladly accepted his invitation to spend the night with him. The next morning after breakfast he gave me a check. I bade him and his family adieu and started on my way back to Brownsville and home. I hadn't gone over ½ the way to Bville when I heard hounds running behind me. I stopped my horse to see whatever they might be chasing when pretty soon a very large deer with large antlers came in sight running parallel with the road and only 20 ft. away. I drew my artillery and loped my horse along by his side and snapped every chamber of those pistols without a single explosion. The deer went safely on his way unless he encountered a more dangerous enemy than I.

I proceeded on my way feeling disgusted and silly, but I learned a lesson here that I have never forgotten: that even in danger pistols sometimes fail to fire. Then they are no protection but may get you into trouble. I went on my way and arrived home safely and handed over those pistols to their owners. I have never carried one since. Had it not been for the lesson I thus learned I would never have written this true incident here.

James W. Crabb's handwritten account, published in Kentucky Explorer, *July–August 2003, provided by Alfred L. Crabb Jr.*

Mose Haney's One-Room School Experience

Mose Haney spent his life attending school and as a teacher in the Carter County school system. He began teaching when he was about twenty years old. His first fifteen years were in a one-room school. During those years he taught at Sutton Branch, Rock Springs, Lower Grassy, Upper Grassy, and Boone Grassy (also known as Boone Furnace or just Boone).

After attending one-room schools near his family's current living location, Mose began his formal education at Christian Normal Institute (now Kentucky Christian University) in Grayson, Carter County. After that he went to Berea College. He lacked money for transportation and college fees, thus worked in the cafeteria to cover costs. He has told how he and his roommate, the late Roscoe Stephens (onetime superintendent of Greenup County Schools), were assigned to clear tables. They were permitted to partake of leftover bread and milk. Consequently, he never liked those foods in later life.

Mose began his one-room teaching experience at Sutton Branch, which was located near his home. At an early age he was known as a firm and caring teacher. He was not much older than some of his students, many of which were relatives from the Haney and Meenach [pronounced Menix] clans.

His next school was Rock Springs, near Gesling, Kentucky, located along Buffalo Creek. Mose and many of his students needed to ford the creek in order to get to school. Some lived near the school, thus didn't have to cross the stream. He was remembered as a young man who influenced many.

Mose was married in 1929 and they lived in the Grassy Creek area. Most of his one-room school teaching time was spent in schools along Grassy Creek. This stream runs through Carter County from near the Lewis County line to join Buffalo Creek. The latter runs into Tygarts near Kehoe, located at the Greenup County line. Three one-room schools occupied the landscape along Grassy Creek. Mose's early years were spent teaching at Lower Grassy, and the school sessions were short. That summer he attended classes at Morehead.

In those days Grassy Creek was a flatbed stream meandering along the way without bridges for crossings. If a person traveled, he/she would have to ford the stream. There was a story, embellished by friends across the years, about Mose's pink long-john underwear. It seems as if he assumed he could drive his old car through the swollen stream. Instead, he had to leave the car and swim to the other side. His burgundy corduroy trousers faded on the union suit–style underwear, making them quite pink. He continued to wear the garments, since times were hard and clothing was scarce.

Eventually, Mose and family moved to Carter City, Kentucky. From there he walked about three miles up a hollow and over a hill to Boone Furnace's one-room school. This school was located along Grassy Creek about midway of the stream's length. He also taught for a couple of years at Upper Grassy, near the Lewis County line.

Mose's one-room school experiences occurred during the mid- to late twenties and thirties. A teacher in a one-room school had a great influence in the community. They had the respect of parents and students. Although Mose attended college for some thirty years, he never earned a degree. At that time a degree was not required. He would always attend classes and add credits to keep his certificate valid. He was always immaculate and neatly dressed. He wore dress shirts, a tie, and what we would today call khakis. There was no permanent press and no electricity in rural Carter County at that time. His wife washed, starched, and ironed his clothes with irons heated on a wood-burning cookstove.

When Franklin D. Roosevelt started the "New Deal" to help the country recover from the Depression, one of the projects was to erect buildings from cut stone. A consolidated school building was constructed at Carter City, Kentucky. When it was completed about 1940–41, Mose was hired as the fifth–sixth grade teacher there. He held this position until his untimely death in October 1955. He had taught for thirty years, with fifteen of them in one-room schools.

Former students praise Mose Haney for his dedication to education and the influence he had on their lives. He would be proud to know that his daughter was a teacher for thirty years, and that some of his grandchildren and great grandchildren are teachers.

Patricia Gibson, daughter of Mose Haney, Greenup, April 11, 2009

RURAL TEACHING

The first one-room school at which I taught was the Mattingly School here in the Loretto area, but it was better known as Frogtown. It was called Frogtown because it was really swampy in that area, and the frogs were plentiful!

I lived at home during the three years I taught there. I traveled to and from school each day in an old touring Chevrolet car. I drove it myself. It had to have curtains put on it if it was raining or bad weather. Otherwise, it was what was called a touring car. The car starter was located inside the car.

One of my favorite memories of being a teacher at the Mattingly School is that I was from the community, so the parents and the children mostly knew me. I really enjoyed my three years there, and the children respected me like I was a queen, and I had boys in school there that were fourteen or fifteen years old. I always called the students from the third grade down "my babies," and I always saw that they were protected.

Students back then never showed any disrespect. It was so different then than what it is like now. We have four daughters in school systems, and they tell me the things children do now that I can't believe.

I enjoyed my teaching years very much. Of course, the number of students varied. I might have three in first grade; maybe two in the second, and so on like that.

I think the number of students I had there each year was thirty-two, except for one year when I had forty-five.

I left Mattingly School after three years because another girl had gone to college and got her two-year degree, and the superintendent moved me and hired her at that school. The superintendent was the boss then! I don't know why he liked her better than he liked me! [*Laughter*] . . .

Upon leaving Mattingly School, I taught [at] Helm School, located about three miles north of Lebanon. Helm was located in an area that had many caves, and one of the caves is seen in one of the photographs that features the students. Not only were caves there, but mounds were there also. They had salt on them, so the deer came there to satisfy their salt needs. They would lick the salt.

I had an honest bunch of school kids during the three years I taught there. I had no problem teaching at any school.

When I taught at Mattingly School, the students were mostly Catholic, but at Helm the religion was mostly a mixture, and at Taylor School where I taught next was non-Catholic.

As a teacher in these rural schools, I was paid sixty-five dollars for each twenty-day school month. The most I ever made was ninety-two dollars for twenty days. The check was monthly, and my record book had to be checked before I received my pay. . . .

The third school at which I taught was Taylor School in Gravel Switch over in the eastern part of Marion County. The students there were really, really nice kids.

The reason I moved from Helm School to Taylor School was because the former teacher at Taylor had been causing trouble. He was a male teacher. The superintendent asked me if I would consider going there to teach and see if I could get things straightened out. I agreed to do it, and everything went really well when I got there. The students there were very respectful.

I taught there for two years, then I got married. Not long after that, I taught for a year at Bringle School in Washington County, and that's the only school where I taught that is still standing.

Mayola Graves, Loretto, September 9, 2008

Teaching Years

The first school at which I taught was Hamilton, located in northern Monroe County, close to Metcalfe. I guess I got that teaching job because my dad worked it out.

I really remember teaching at Rock Bridge School, because you [the author], your brother Charles, and Wallace McGuire went to school there. I haven't seen Wallace since then, and I don't think he's living now.

On the first day at Hamilton, when you wanted to get a drink of water, you had to hold up your hand and stand up on the floor if you wanted to go get a drink.

I remember one little boy who, instead of a penny pencil, had a better grade of a pencil. It was Yellow Number 2, leaded. He felt like he was rich when he started to school, and he had that pencil stuck in his overalls' bib pocket!

All total, I taught one-room schools known as Hamilton, Rock Bridge, Merryville, Oak Hill, and Union Hill.

Mamie Wright, Tompkinsville, October 16, 2008

Portraits of Buckeye and Fourmile

The first one-room school at which I taught was called Buckeye. It was in Carter County, a few miles from Grayson, in a location called Pactolus. I drove an old Chevy station wagon part of the way. I parked at a small grocery store owned by May Webster, then joined students in walking across the Little Sandy Bridge. The bridge bottom was full of holes, and parents requested that the teacher walk with students to supervise their safety. Several students lived on the side of the river where the school was located, and met us there.

Buckeye was a wonderful little school. Parents and the community were dedicated to the students' educational accomplishments. Students were obedient and respectful of others and the teacher.

In the white, wood building, a potbelly stove occupied the center. A long bench was near the front, facing the blackboard. This was known as the recitation bench. In turn, each class would come forward to the bench for reading, recitation, and instruction. Others continued to do seat work at the same time. Older students often helped the younger ones, and assisted me by writing assignments on the board. We had no way to make copies of seat work other than some workbooks. Materials were scarce, but we used resources to the fullest.

I felt successful, and truly enjoyed my first year of teaching. The following year I was replaced and sent to another school farther away. My replacement was more advanced toward her degree, and her family was a firm supporter of the superintendent and the school administration. That is the way it was in Carter County in 1956. . . .

The physical aspect of the Fourmile School, at which I taught, was truly a handicap. The building was constructed on a hillside with one side at ground level, and the other jacked up on pillars. There was very little space to play. A neighboring farmer came to school one day complaining that the students were getting on his grassland. There was no fence, no boundary line, etc.; my students just had to be careful. There was no place to practice relay races and other activities for the annual school fair. Outdoor activities had to be restricted to games not requiring a lot of space.

A lunchroom [kitchen] had been established and occupied a room which had been added to the main room. This was an interruption because all traffic to the kitchen had to go through the main classroom. There was no running water, so a lot of water carrying took place.

It was my job to bring groceries to supplement the government commodities. Perhaps the nourishment was enough to warrant the lunchroom business.

That was a very unsettling year for me, so I was pleased to be transferred to another location.

Patricia Gibson, Greenup, April 11, 2009

Teaching in a Remote School

The Bull Creek one-room school is located in southeastern Kentucky in Letcher County. The school building was built by hand by two local men, Will Haynes and Morgan Sexton. It is approximately three and one-half miles east of Cornetesville, and three miles west of Carcassonne. It sits on a small area of ground with a creek nearby, and beside a one-lane dirt road. The road was barely usable by automobiles. The mail was usually delivered by horseback.

The school opened for classes in 1946. The building is one large room with a coal- and wood-burning stove on the right side. The cloakroom was a place where the students could put their coats, hats, and lunch when they arrived each morning. There was no inside bathroom, but there was an outhouse out back.

During the winter months one or two boys would come early in the morning and build a fire in the potbelly stove. The room would be nice and warm when other students and the teacher arrived. A variety of teachers came and went at the school. Some of them stayed only one year. There were seven different teachers during the eleven years the school was open. Many of the teachers boarded with Will and Catherine Haynes, who lived about one mile from the school. The teachers walked to school from there. Teachers were hard to find because of the remote location and poor roads.

My tenure at the school began in January 1956, when I was a senior at Stuart Robinson High School, which is located in the community of Letcher in Letcher County. My father, Clifton Caudill, heard that the teacher at the Bull Creek School had left at Christmas and would not be returning due to her ill health. My father knew the county school superintendent, Arlie Boggs, so he asked Mr. Boggs if he would consider hiring me to finish out the year. He explained that he knew that was a very unusual request. Mr. Boggs said he would think about it. My father explained my situation to him as well.

I was taking classes one-half the day and working in the administrative offices in the afternoon. That was to earn money I needed for my graduation and other expenses. I only needed one more credit to have what I needed to graduate, and the others could be dropped. I had a relative in the accounting class that I would continue with. She lived near the school where I would be teaching and could bring my assignments home to me each day and then return them to the teacher. The high school teacher had agreed to this plan. After some consideration, Mr. Boggs decided to let me teach the rest of the year since it probably would be impossible to find someone on such short notice, especially during winter.

I was very excited about getting the job and making ninety-four dollars a month. I thought I would be rich! I was also anxious about the first day on the job and wondering what lay ahead for me. Many of the students were my relatives, so I questioned whether this would be a better or worse situation. I lived at Carcassonne, about three miles from the school.

That first morning was a cold winter day. I packed my lunch and struck out early to walk the three miles. My mind was racing with thoughts as to what I was getting into. When I arrived I was greeted by a young boy who had made a nice warm fire. The heat felt wonderful and welcoming since I was very cold from the long walk.

The other students began to come in. I felt sure they also had questions about what was going to happen at school. There were twelve of these students, ranging in ages [from] seven to fourteen, and grades 2 through 8. Many of them were related—brothers, sisters, and cousins. Everyone walked to school most of the time even though they may have lived several miles away. We spent most of the day getting better acquainted. We also looked at their textbooks and tried to determine what grade each child was in. Some of the 1 through 8 grades had no students. There were students in grades 2, 3, 4, 6, and 8.

During that first day the students told me they had not spent much time studying on school lessons this year. They had done some spelling, reading, and math. They said they had spent a lot of time playing games. Their favorite was marbles. They also said that when recess is over, I should ring the big bell and boys and girls would line up on separate lines.

I quickly realized that I had my work cut out for me. We divided up their books and tried to decide where to begin. Through trial and error we eventually worked out a system. We decided to try combining some of the lessons and teach two grade levels together. With just two or three students in each grade, this worked out. We combined some grade 2 and 3 subjects. We also tried some grade 4 and 6 subjects with the sixth-grade students helping the younger ones with their reading and math. One advantage to a one-room school is that the students can learn from each other by listening to what others are being taught. Little ears perk up when they hear something that interests them.

Shelby Jean Caudill, Madisonville, September 25, 2009

Teaching at Sugar Grove

The name of the one-room school at which I first taught was Sugar Grove, located in Magan, Ohio County, on Sunnydale Road. Basically, I rode a horse to school every day because I didn't have an automobile. I had thirty-one students, grades 1 through 8. I laughingly tell people that I likely learned more than the students did! We had an old recitation bench, as it was called back then. I'd call a class up and use that recitation bench for what we called "hearing a class" back then.

We had an old potbelly stove, and it was a big job to keep the stovepipe in. We had no running water except when the roof leaked. We had privy houses on the outside, one for the boys and one for the girls.

We had five erasers and one chalkboard that was falling down.

All the students brought their lunch in a little molasses bucket, and they put it in the cloakroom where they hung their heavy clothes during winter months.

At noon we had an hour off. We played by who, fox and dogs, and other games. I was their teacher, but I played right along with them.

We had a bucket and a chain, both of which were used to draw water from the old well, and everyone drank out of the same bucket.

I made $68.20 per month for teaching, and that school year only lasted seven months.

I was single then, lived at home, and rode a horse to school every day. I built a little pole pen with a shed on it to keep my horse during school hours.

That's the way things were back then. . . .

I remember very well when I told the students there at Sugar Grove School that today would be my last day. When I said that, there wasn't a dry eye in the room, including myself. I always thought that I did some of the best teaching in that one-room school than anywhere else. You had to work hard at it.

A lot of those students went on to high school, and some of them turned out real well, educationally and financially wise. It's sad to say that many of those students have passed away.

Noble H. Midkiff, Whitesville, December 1, 2008

Teaching at White Oak

During the last of May 1947, I worked two weeks down here as a waitress at the Corner Restaurant. My mother said to me, "I've got you a ride to Lindsey-Wilson College. You're going to ride with Smith Edwards in his pickup truck every day to Lindsey, and you're going to be a teacher."

So I did what Mama said. I rode back and forth with Smith Edwards until he got through with that—fall, winter, spring. I got me a sleeping room in Columbia. So I was a sophomore, age nineteen, when I began teaching at White Oak, a one-room school.

I taught the full school year at White Oak. School started in July, took off one day for Thanksgiving, one or two days for Christmas, and it was dismissed the last of January.

When school was turned out, I started in the spring semester at Lindsey, and graduated in 1949 there at Lindsey.

I was paid $96 each month for teaching there at White Oak, but had to pay the taxi $30! See, I had to ride a taxi from Edmonton to White Oak, and then the driver came to get me each afternoon. However, lots of times he would forget me, and I'd walk halfway back to Edmonton before he would remember me. But he still charged me the same $30.

The Metcalfe County sheriff was the owner of the taxi, and that was the deal—$30 each month. The sheriff had a sawmill and one taxi as his personal business property.

There were about seventeen children at the White Oak School, and they were all kinfolks. One of the boys was the only one in seventh grade. His name was Dallas Roosevelt Wilson, and he was an uncle to some of the other students and cousins to the rest of them. All that family revolved around the Wilsons. His daddy was Sherman Wilson and he was a big politician, so everybody looked up to him.

Dallas Roosevelt Wilson is the one who built the fires for me every day. I never built a fire in my life. We would have frozen if he hadn't built the fires every day. And he's the one that took me to all the homes in the neighborhood, because we had to walk and visit everybody and fill out lots of papers about all the kids at home—their birthdays, when they'd be going to school, and other things. We had all that paperwork to do. I believe that was another man's job in the education building. I forget his title, but he was the one that was supposed to go around to see who would be coming to school next year. But we had to do what he was supposed to do.

That was after school was dismissed in the afternoon. Dallas would walk with me to these homes to fill out the papers. One home was two miles away; some were close, and some were a good ways off. I don't know what I would have done without Dallas. At that time he was fifteen and I was nineteen. . . .

There wasn't a chalkboard in the White Oak school building, but a space was painted black on the wall, and that was what we used for a blackboard. And I didn't have a bookshelf, so my mama, who could do most anything, took orange crates and nailed them together, then painted them dark green. What she made was a stand-up bookcase. She also took some little nail kegs and made some chairs for the little kids to use when they sat down to hear me teaching them to read. She painted them green to match the bookcase, made some little pillows to go on them, and they looked pretty. . . .

To get water for White Oak School, it was way, way over the hill. They had to walk through a part of the woods and way over a big hill to get to the spring. The boys were the ones that went to get a bucket of water. I didn't use the same boys each time; they rotated.

We had to have a little drinking cup or, if they didn't have a cup, they had to make one out of paper. They'd fold the paper to make a little cup. Each student had their own cup. We had a dipper that was used to get the water from the bucket, but each student had to drink from their own cup.

I've still got my little drinking cup at home.

Billie Sue Blakeman, Edmonton, September 22, 2008

TEACHING IN A SECLUDED SCHOOL

After two years at Western Kentucky College, I went back to Trimble County and taught at Norfork School in 1938–39. While teaching there, I stayed at home and drove my grandfather's car to school. I made $52.50 each month while teaching there for seven months.

I lived only a few miles from there, but it was a secluded area and I was not familiar with it, but it was in the north part of Trimble County. The school nurse made visits out through the county in those days to take care of sick people.

Before school started, I went with her and we visited several of the homes of the children who were going to be coming to Norfork School. I can remember walking across a creek! It was just a very rural area. I think the school was named after Northfork Creek, which may have run into Corn Creek.

There was a road that cut through to the top of river hill, down the hill, and through that creek area, and then on up to the town of Bedford.

When school started, I was new to it, and the students were new to me, but they were very receptive and kind. I had about thirty-eight children in that school, seventeen of whom were in first and second grade, and one in eighth grade. I think I had students in all grades except the sixth. The seventeen in first and second grade was a real challenge!

My big challenge there was teaching an eighth grader in a class by herself to be able to take the test, because in those days you still had to go take a test in the county seat in order to pass. It was just a challenge to present enough information to a class that small. She moved away from that school before the school year was out, but she made her grade.

She didn't seem very excited in class each day, but she was patient.

Virginia DeBoe, Eddyville, October 7, 2008

LIFE AND TIMES AT SCHOOL BACK THEN

The thing I always thought about this one-room school was that you were not only the teacher, you were also the custodian, cook, and everything. But what we did was hire boys to build the fire. I remember paying one boy, who was a student, ten cents a day for building the fire, and he would have the building nice and warm when we got there. You couldn't do that today, but we did it then because parents allowed it.

Parents would allow us to bring the kids home with us around Christmastime. I wasn't married at the time, so I stayed with my mom and dad. So at Christmastime I'd bring a couple of boys home with me, give them their own room there at home and let them help us pack the treat. Treats consisted of maybe an orange, an apple, and maybe a bar of candy. That was really kind of special to them.

One thing I always thought about the one-room school was that you knew everybody. Everybody knew you, and you knew every student by name, and knew all the parents. If you had a problem, all you had to do was stop and tell the parent about it, or send word to them, and they'd be there next day.

I don't remember having a serious problem, but kids would smoke occasionally, just tobacco such as Old North State and Prince Albert. They also smoked what was called Rabbit Everlasting, something that grew up in the fields around there. The girls would tell on the boys when the smoke was coming out of the boys' toilet! I don't remember any of the girls smoking. And the boys chewed a little tobacco also.

Those kids were truly good kids. I didn't have a lot of problems with them.

I didn't fuss at them for smoking, but I tried to tell them that smoking wasn't good for them.

Bige R. Warren, Barbourville, November 20, 2008

TEACHING AT PENICK

I began teaching at Penick in 1948, after one year of college at Western. I applied for a teaching job at Penick, and I think it was a school for which they had some trouble getting a teacher since it was kind of in a back area. It wasn't very far off Highway 80, but a lot of people didn't know where Penick was. But I did, because I grew up down there.

The funniest thing was that when I started teaching there, I wanted the kids to call me Miss Frazier, which was my maiden name. Those kids thought that was the funniest thing that ever was, so they said, "We're not going to call you that; you are Virginia."

They all knew me!

I said, "Say 'Miss Virginia.'" And they finally got to where they called me that, and that stuck to me all the years of my teaching. I was always Miss Virginia. Even now, when I walk down the street here in Edmonton, I'll hear people holler, "Hello, Miss Virginia!" [*Laughter*]

I may hear them say to someone, "Miss Virginia was my second grade teacher." . . .

The first school in which I taught was Penick School, and I actually went to school there until I was in fifth grade, and my daddy's family went there to that school also. Most of his family members went on and made teachers, but my dad was the only one that didn't. The ones that taught then went on and worked at other things later on. One of my uncles taught there when I was in school.

Virginia Janes, Edmonton, September 22, 2008

A LOT OF FIRST GRADERS

When I began teaching at Missouri Hollow I had forty-seven students, but sixteen of them were in first grade. The first grade was hard to get kids started, because we didn't have kindergarten back then. Thus, first grade was usually harder than the others because you had to get them used to coming to school, to get them ready for school. I guess my most difficult class was first grade, because the problem was being able to get them started doing schoolwork.

Why I had so many first graders at that time was because we were not allowed to socially promote students. They had to come to school so many days out of the school year so they could get their work com-

pleted before you could promote them to the next grade. School was
not compulsory at this time, so some of the students who had to walk
a long ways would only come the first few months of school while the
weather was pretty. You didn't see them anymore that year. That meant
you could have teenagers in first grade, which I did.

I used seventh- and eighth-grade students to help me, like when I
would teach something in the first and second grade, even third. I would
let these older students work with younger students while I went ahead
and taught the fifth- and sixth-grade students. So what I did was use the
upper grades to help me with the lower grades. I did that all the time.

Wanda Humble, Monticello, November 7, 2008

TEACHING IN ONE-ROOM SCHOOLS' FINAL YEARS

I began teaching in one-room schools, first at Bryant School, located in
the Sano community. The school had burned down, and they replaced
it with a new block building a year or two before I got there. I taught
there for four years. The first year I taught there I had forty students
during the year, twelve of whom were first graders. I was twenty years
old when I started teaching there, but before I started there my husband and I went over and visited all the homes in which we could find
people at home. They were good neighbors, the very best place one
would ever want to teach.

After four years I looked around and these students going into fifth
hadn't had another teacher for four years. They didn't want me to move
away, and I didn't want to move, but I thought it best for the students.
At that point in time, the county was beginning to close the one-room
schools, so I taught one year at Maple Grove in Milltown, Adair County.
It was also a one-room school, and I had thirty-some students there. I
taught there for only one year, then had a new baby.

The superintendent then said, "If you'll take Tabernacle School
located in Dunnville, Adair County, near Casey County, so we'll have a
qualified teacher in it, I'll hire a substitute." He went on to say, "I'll give
you your sick leave time, so you won't have to set foot in that school." I
took sick leave, and had a sub who taught until sometime in February,
then I went back. I only had twelve students at Tabernacle. I paid in my
retirement, so I got a full year's credit.

Then I taught a one-year at Conover School, which is off Highway
80. That was also a good school. That year the school board decided

all the one-room schools had to prepare lunch for their students. The county furnished the food and they gave us a refrigerator, but we had to cook the food on a potbelly stove. The milkman brought the milk, and the bread man brought the bread. Once a month we'd have to go pick up our supplies for the whole month, and I put them here at home in the kitchen, because you couldn't leave them at school. If you did somebody might steal them. So each day I had to take the food that we were going to cook that day at school. That only lasted one year.

Zona Royse, Columbia, October 4, 2008

VERY MODEST SALARY

My salary was $63.60 per month. My dad bought a 1937 Ford car that replaced a Model T we had. Well, I had to pay about $42 per month on that car, so that's why I had to borrow money to go back to school.

I got one dollar a month more for my salary my second year, and a dollar more for my third year, but sometimes the money wasn't even there at the end of the month. That's how great the Depression was. But I'd get my money on Monday, or the next Friday.

Marguerite Wilson, Leitchfield, October 1, 2008

TEACHING THE SPARKSES

There was a carpool at the time I was teaching at Granny Richardson Springs School in Estill County, and we had a man who was hauling me and three other teachers. He charged just $1 each day to transport us. In my case he let me out at the top of the hill, then I had to walk down a long, winding road down to the bottom of this hill to the Granny Richardson Springs School. My first paycheck was $118.30 each month, so after I paid my car-riding bill I had about $100 left. That driver taught at a two-room school on top of that mountain, known as Barnes Mountain. The second year at that same school I had my own car, so I got to be the driver. My salary during the third year was $157 per month. That was a pretty good increase.

I had twelve students at that school, and most of them belonged to Eli Sparks, who had a big home on a hill there by the school. He operated a sawmill that was located right there, and an oil well. At least one of the oil wells was owned by the school, so they got royalty from it. In that instance, I was told that they had some advantages that the other students didn't have. I didn't know what the advantages were at the time.

Anyway, one-half the students were his children. Two of them were daughters, twelve or thirteen years old, which was close to my age.

Maryanna Barnes, Frankfort, October 14, 2008

First Experiences

I was scared the first day when I went to teach at Davis Bend. I didn't like to talk in front of people. We started out with the primer class, but I was so disappointed that I wanted to go on to second grade or something. But before then I had to take the first grade.

We had three or four different kinds of school buildings in the county. One kind was just plain weather-boarded, which was the kind I attended. We also had cobblestone buildings made out of natural rocks, and we had brick. The one I taught at Davis Bend was built with brick, and the one I attended as a kid was weather-boarded. It had big high ceilings in it. Somebody had to bring in wood and coal, but we did get water from a hand pump. We were a little ahead of the rest of the schools with that pump.

Under the schoolhouse there was a big hole, and we could store wood and coal and other things. Well, hogs would get under the schoolhouse and would root and holler during school. And dogs would get into fights. Lots of things like that happened. We also didn't have a stock law, so cows would run around the schoolhouse, and they slept in the ball field right at the foot of the hill.

My cousin came down from up north and enrolled there. He jumped on that old cow's back and that cow took him around the hillsides!

We had some good experiences there. . . .

My first day of teaching was pretty interesting. I had thirty-eight students in all eight grades, and they had run two or three teachers away from that school. Those kids had no rules, no nothing.

This was in a little brick school building located up on a hill. It had a stove in the middle of the floor and had a pump where we got our water.

I was licensed in secondary education and had to get an emergency elementary certificate to teach there, but I was lucky to just get a job. At that time there weren't many jobs available.

I rode the school bus part of the way out there and walked the rest of the way.

During bad days the school bus didn't go very far, so I'd walk about a mile all the way around the river bluff back on the hill.

When I first started teaching I guess I learned more than the kids did that first year. They were used to chewing tobacco, so I got all their tobacco and put it in my desk drawer. It made me sick just sitting there smelling it.

The older girls liked to read true stories. They'd bring a magazine and sit down and read it. So I had to make rules, had to put boundary lines to keep them on the school grounds. Some of them were used to going down in the fields and some down towards the river. So I made rules as to the school ground boundary and enforced them.

Pat McDonald, Barbourville, November 21, 2008

Early Days

I graduated from Knox Central High School in 1948. That summer my oldest sister, Mae, was taking classes at Union College. I also took two courses, a total of seven hours, at that time. During the winter of that year, the children had run a teacher off at Bull Creek–Sprule School.

My dad heard about it, and since I had seven hours of college work the superintendent said I could teach on an emergency certificate. I arranged to stay with an old lady whose husband worked away from home from Monday through Thursday night.

At that school I only had seventeen students. I taught as I had been taught. Our only A.V. [audiovisual] materials were our textbooks and a flag. The children brought their paper, pencils, and crayons if they had any. Our daily routine was from 8:00 until 2:30 or 3:00 p.m. We began the day with the pledge of allegiance to the flag. Then someone would read a verse or two from the Bible. We had reading, which was assigned the day before, and students took turns reading orally. After that we had discussion, spelling, and then recess, math, and lunch, of which the children brought to school in a metal pail or a brown paper bag. We had English, then afternoon recess, and then either geography or history until time to go home.

On Friday afternoon we had either a spelling bee or an adding match.

I always participated in outside games such as ante over, ring around the roses, drop the handkerchief, hide and go seek, or whoopee-hide, and ball games.

If it were too bad to go outside, we played "I see something with my little eye and the color of it is ——." Whoever guessed right was "it" the next time. We also played red rover, red rover. If it snowed one student, whose name was Kenneth, brought a homemade sled and we all took turns sliding down a little hill that was conveniently located at the edge of the playground.

Laura Agnes Townsley Stacy, Barbourville, November 21, 2008

TEACHING IN THE EARLY YEARS

The first school at which I taught was at Verona, here in Boone County. It was a one-room school located at the top of Houston Hill. The desks were a small table and chair in which the students sat, and mine was just like theirs. The kids' desk also had an inkwell on the top right side, and the back of one desk was attached to the top of the next one. There were twenty students present that year, and most of them were from farm families.

For heat we had a potbelly stove in the middle of the room.

I boarded weekly with the Cravens family, and paid them $5 per week. My monthly salary at that time was $35.50.

In 1918 women teachers wore only dresses to school, and that's the way I dressed.

Since Verona was a one-room school, I taught all subjects in all grades. The basic courses were reading, writing, spelling, arithmetic, history, geography, and I taught physiology to the upper grades.

Students there at Verona were good-behaving children, but there were a few that would have to be corrected.

When the new Verona School was built, I taught there with Ava Lou Hudson Walton, my friend across the years. . . .

The second school at which I taught was East Bend, which was located near where the CG&E power plant is located. CG&E is now called Duke Power Plant.

We lived directly across the Ohio River from East Bend at Piet's Landing. My father or my brother would take me across the river in the morning and come after me in the afternoon. The boat they used was a fishing boat that was called a John boat. Another kind of boat they sometimes used was a skift [skiff], which was a little better boat.

East Bend School was much larger than the one at Verona, and I had forty-five students.

All students walked to school back then, as their parents didn't take them. School years back then lasted eight months. While teaching there I boarded with the Charles Bodie family.

The county soon had a new building built by my father and Mr. Craven, and it was named Hume School. It was located at the foot of Houston Hill by Green Mountain ballpark. That building is still standing and is used as a residence.

While I was teaching there the room was large enough to have a place to cook on one side. It was used as a cooking class. It was for the future, something we thought was coming at that time. However, consolidation came and the rural schools were soon gone,

There was an older boy in school there, and each cold morning he would get there early and build a fire. I boarded with the Lon Wilson family while teaching at Hume School.

All one-room schools in the 1920s had outside bathroom facilities. There wasn't running water anywhere.

Told by Agnes Chandler Kenney, Walton, May 8, 1988, to Kathleen Wiley

Green behind the Ears

The first day of school at Goble Branch, all twelve students came and looked at a nineteen-year-old "green behind the ears" teacher. Those twelve students began the process of teaching me more than I would ever teach them.

I had two years of college at Morehead, but ran out of money and decided to go home to Prestonsburg and try to get hired on at the Kentucky–West Virginia Gas Company. I was placed on their waiting list. That summer my stepmother, who worked for the Floyd County Board of Education, was in charge of schoolbooks. She heard about Goble Branch School and that nobody wanted to walk two miles in and two miles out every day. I was happy to get a job and later very thankful to have found a profession that I loved, so I spent thirty-seven years working with boys and girls.

Goble Branch School was closed for good at the end of the 1959–1960 school year. . . .

The first time I looked at the building, I could see it was about twenty feet by forty feet, and was painted white. The school had one front door, and to reach it you climbed up five concrete steps.

Inside the building it had wood floors which had been oiled. There were twenty old desks, and there were bench seats at the front of each desk. Each desktop had room for two students to place their pencils in two groups. (At present I have one of those desks in my living room.)

In the middle of the room was a potbelly stove with a stovepipe going up through the ceiling. I later paid a student fifteen cents a week to build a fire each morning. Occasionally too much coal was put in the stove and the stovepipe became red. When that happened I opened the door and left it open until cooling took place. Coal was stored under the building, as the building was built five feet above ground.

I haven't thought about this for fifty years!

Thomas "Rube" Tackett, Prestonsburg, December 6, 2008

Two Minutes to Teach

When I was teaching at Farmers Chapel here in Taylor County, it was a large school, and I was a young teacher only nineteen years old. The country schools were not too far apart, so there was another school just a little ways over. There were some children that lived on the line between Farmers Chapel and Jones Chapel, and they heard there was a new teacher coming to Farmers. They were allowed to go to either school, so they all decided to come to Farmers just to see what I was like.

I had only forty-one students at Farmers, and here come the others one day. In those days student teaching didn't amount to much. Well, what I did was to pattern my school days like it was when I was a student in a one-room school.

I figured out one day [that with] all the classes for which I was responsible, I had only about two minutes each day to do those classes. In those days the thing about it was that the older students helped you an awful lot. Well, I had a really good seventh grade that year, and they weren't an awful lot younger than I was.

All country schools back in those days had to have a box supper, and that school certainly needed the money. We had cloth over the windows when I first went there. We had to put wood under the floor. The school was not in good shape. I told my superintendent, "You know what, you did that to me in order to see if I was made out of the right stuff." Well, I reckon I was, because I stayed with it thirty-five years.

Betty Garner Williams, Campbellsville, December 11, 2008

Teaching at McClendon

I taught my first year in a one-room school. That was in 1947, and to get there I rode a horse to and from school. I did not complete that year of teaching. In 1948 I taught all eight grades at McClendon School in northern Wayne County. I continued teaching there until 1964, at which time there were too few students, due to this portion of the county being secluded by the coming of Lake Cumberland.

While teaching at McClendon, this was a stable community and some students were with me during all eight grades. As roads improved, pupils were at first transported by private vehicle to Nancy High School, located in Pulaski County.

Children walked to and from McClendon School each day, some for at least two miles; others closer. Water was carried from a nearby spring to drink, and used to wash our hands, clean windows, and scrub desks and floors, as needed.

There was a long, rectangular, log-burning stove at first, then it was replaced by a round, potbelly, coal-burning stove. I think we did eventually get electricity, but I'm not sure. . . .

I enjoyed my teaching years at McClendon, and the students seemed to really appreciate me. On June 9, 2007, these former students had a reunion in my honor. Since the school building no longer exists, the reunion was held in the home of one of my former students, Doris Decker Hubbard. All of them seemed appreciative of their experiences at school.

Betty Holmes McClendon, Nancy, December 16, 2008

Teaching in a Secluded Area

The only person I know that taught in a one-room school and is still living is my brother, whose name is V. C. Midkiff. He is a retired chemist from the University of Kentucky. He taught his first school in Breckenridge County during the fall 1939, in a little community called Buras.

My brothers and I went up there and played a little country music, and we went up there on a Saturday and played for a little party. We had to open seven gates on a county road in order to get into that area. My brother boarded there with some old people that ran a little country store. He, too, has many memories of the Buras community back in 1939, where he taught his first and only one-room school.

Noble H. Midkiff, Whitesville, December 1, 2008

"Primitive" Conditions; Good Students

Upon arriving at Fairview School in cooler weather, "Job One" was to crank up the central heating system, a modern state-of-the-art piece of equipment that operated without electricity. This was fortunate because there was no electricity in the school.

This masterful piece of equipment that supported creature comfort was a potbelly stove that sat in the middle of the room. I always had to make sure that there was enough dry kindling and coal on hand. And don't forget the matches!

Some percentage of the students, twenty-six of them, were always too hot or too cold, depending on the weather and their location relative to the stove. They were given permission for a wide range of movement to permit them to stay reasonably comfortable.

They were a hearty group and very rarely did they complain about conditions which, by today's standards, bordered on primitive.

After getting the fire going, the next job was to get drinking water for our "cooler" from a well near the south side of the building. The health department had earlier sited our two outhouses on the north side of the school for obvious reasons. For those persons who do not know about an outhouse, it was a very basic, slit trench toilet, complete with a half-moon on the door, and occasionally with an old Sears and Roebuck catalog, not necessarily used for reading purposes! It was a real adventure to use these facilities in the winter. Since we had no running water, we always put a bucket of water and a dipper near the door for hand washing.

The health department required that our water "cooler" have several drops of bleach put in it to kill any germs. The kids didn't use bleach in the water at home and really despised its taste. On more than one occasion, when I was otherwise distracted, fresh water would surreptitiously be substituted. I don't know of any harm this caused. . . .

Classes at Fairview would start with the pledge of allegiance, which was recited by all, including the first graders. The order of classes varied from day to day. Some of my older students helped with the younger ones when possible. I was indeed fortunate that nearly all of the students were very capable in their studies so that I could teach the classes and not have to spend an inordinate time on an individual.

Separate time was reserved for special instruction so that other students could work on something else. The students were well mannered and nondisruptive, unlike some of the town school students. I am most proud of the fact that I had no disciplinary issues at school. Most kids were hard workers in school and at home. Many had to miss school to help with the crops, particularly during tobacco season. Unfortunately, some had to continue working at home after they completed the eighth grade and did not continue on to high school. . . .

We did not have a flagpole at Fairview when I started teaching. With the help of several of the students (some of them were stronger than I was), this situation was soon corrected. We located a suitable pine tree, cut it down and removed the bark. After it dried a little we painted it white, dug a hole, and erected it in front of the school. Everyone showed a lot of pride in our accomplishment. They knew what respect of the flag meant.

The school system did not have a budget for this sort of thing, so I bought the paint, flag, and other materials. I was making $110 base pay per month and this seemed a lot more money than I was making at my previous summer job, where I earned 25¢ per hour washing dishes in the school cafeteria. I guess the pay per hour wasn't that much more but it seemed like it since I stayed at home and did not have to pay that expensive tuition.

Many of the teachers took classes at night in town to get additional college credits and subsequently more pay. One noteworthy class, Kentucky History, required that we memorize the 120 counties and their county seats, not an easy task for the older teachers.

William H. Nicholls Jr., The Villages, Fla., December 14, 2008

QUITE UNPREPARED BY COLLEGE

In 1965 I was offered a job in Morgan County teaching in a one-room school with all grades, first through eighth. The school was named Peddler Gap after a peddler that was murdered and robbed near the school site. Roads in the area were narrow, bridges bad and too dangerous for bus transportation.

I had graduated from college and was in desperate need of a job. I had no clue as to how to teach, and certainly not all grades 1 through

8. My job description from the superintendent was brief. I would get to school by carpooling with two other teachers that taught in other one-room schools in that same area. He suggested that they would help me and answer any questions I had. Thankfully, they were very helpful.

I was excited to pick up my supplies for the new year. I was issued a coal bucket, shovel, water bucket, dipper, box of chalk, six erasers, and a redbird book for keeping attendance and student information. These were considered to be the needed supplies for the school year.

When I arrived the first day of school, forty students and parents were waiting to greet me. I knew my college classes had not prepared me for what was in store. The children ranged in age from six to fifteen, and the majority of them came from four families. Fifteen, twelve, ten, and eight were the number of children in those four families. The children's names rhymed: Connie, Monnie, Donnie, Vonnie, Ronnie, and so on. Their names were hard for me to keep straight.

The school was an early 1900s building made of wood by parents of the children in the neighborhood. The county furnished $190 for the building materials. The ceilings were high and dark. A coal-burning potbelly stove was located in the center of the thirty-by-fifty-[feet] room, and it came in handy when the weather got cold. Summers were extremely hot and the newly oiled floors had a very pungent odor, but it did keep down dust. The seats were bench seats that seated two students and had book storage under the desktop.

Since my college method courses had not covered how to have classes in all subjects for eight grades, I solved this problem by placing the smaller children in bench seats with the larger students, who subsequently helped them with their reading, writing, and math.

Jimmie Jones, West Liberty, December 28, 2008

FAIR-WEATHER TEACHING

The one-room school at which I taught was Walnut Hill School in Metcalfe County, and I had approximately twenty students. Most of them walked to school. A few of them who lived greater distance away from school were brought in cars by their parents My daddy and mama sacrificed the family car in order for me to have transportation. I drove approximately six miles each way. During those years school began in July and ended in early January, therefore escaping the bad weather in January and February.

My salary was $68 and some cents each month

I really had a pleasant year of teaching and I cannot honestly say that there were difficult times during the day. During the really cold weather, getting to school and getting the fire started was somewhat of a task because it took some time for the room to warm.

I had three children who were slow learners to a great degree for their chronological age. We also did not compete with other schools in sports. Games were played in and around the school in our own schoolyard.

Nell S. Eaton, Glasgow, January 8, 2009

DISCOVERING A CALLING

It was purely by coincidence that I got into the teaching profession. In late August of 1971 my younger sister was approached about the possibility of teaching the first two weeks at a small school located on the far side of the county while the regular teacher completed her recovery from surgery. My sister was not all that interested but hated to turn down a good friend.

I was next in line. My oldest son was in school, and the other one soon to follow. My parents and grandparents lived nearby and were more than willing to help out. The thirty-minute early morning trip across the ridge and up a hollow was to change my life.

The first morning on the first day of school was an eye-opener for all concerned. The regular teacher at school had taught this particular group of children and their older brothers and sisters for the past number of years. I was the only stranger. The small group of students, numbering about fifteen, ranged from age six to perhaps ten. Some parents were there the first morning to inquire about "Mrs. Rena's health" and be assured that she would be back by the next week.

Mrs. Rena had used her recovery time well; she had made [school-work] packets for every child and had specific instructions for each student. I was simply there to make sure the schedule was followed. At about 11:00 each morning I would look at the posted menu, pick out the listed cans, and heat up the meal for the day. After quietly eating their lunch, the children would slip outside to play around the door while I tidied up the small kitchen area. In the afternoon they would complete more assignments and I would read aloud to them until it was time to go home. That was our quiet, orderly daily routine.

Teaching there was my introduction to the close communities and the painfully shy children who still populated our county, and to children and schoolhouses that reminded me so much of my own early years in a one-room school. When I was asked by the county administration if I would be willing to substitute in the other rural schools, I said yes.

Norma Ramsey Eversole, Mt. Vernon, January 5, 2009

CITY OF MARION'S FIRST BLACK SCHOOL

In 1926 the Marion, Kentucky, school board built a one-room school building for the black children on North Weldon Street at the edge of town. The school was called Rosenwald and included grades 1 through 8. Miss Laffie Colefield was the first teacher, and Miss Vena Colefield followed her.

In 1930 the board began planning to provide transportation and tuition for the graduates to attend high school in neighboring Caldwell County. A bus was purchased in 1936 to transport the high school children to Princeton.

The first bus driver was Rev. Burns, a black man who could not get insurance because he was black. Wilfred Drake took over as driver until the fall of 1955 when five Rosenwald students entered Marion High School. Rosenwald was closed in 1965 and their students entered into Marion city schools.

Anna Smith Collins, Marion, November 20, 2008

TEACHING AT MITCHELL RUN

In the summer of 1947, our Superintendent of Spencer County Schools came to my home and told me that there was a need for a teacher in a rural school on Salt River, Mitchell Run, several miles from where I was living. He was encouraging, saying that I had been a very good student in high school and if I would take two correspondence courses during the year, I would be issued an emergency certificate for that school year.

I was overwhelmed! What did I know about teaching? I had only played school with younger children. As the story continues, I accepted the challenge. I had 18 students at the beginning of the year in grades 1–8.

We began each day with a Bible reading, the pledge of allegiance to the flag, and singing "America." Since I lacked experience, I modeled my teaching strategy after the teacher who had taught me in the two-room grade school that I had attended. Instruction began with putting the assignments on the blackboard for the upper grades. I then began with the first grade, teaching ABC's and reading with the children. I usually spent about 15 minutes with each group. If the older students finished their work, they could help the younger children, which was easy for all of us. Each class learned from the others.

Everyone had to listen and think while I explained a new process or concept. There were usually one to five pupils in a grade, so it was easy for the students to help each other and still have time to help the younger ones.

Very few books were available and not many supplies, only what I provided. Each child had a set of books for his grade, reading, spelling, arithmetic, history, language and geography. Almost all the children had pencils, tablets and crayons. . . .

The children brought their lunch to school in a lunch box or a paper bag. Water was brought in from the well that was in the corner of the schoolyard. We also had two outhouses, one for the boys and one for the girls located in opposite directions. There was also a coalhouse near the side of the building. The coal was used to heat our room that had a pot-bellied stove in the center.

I was not just the teacher, I was also the nurse, counselor, janitor and whatever else was required to meet the needs of the children. About once a month, the children and I would oil the wooden floor with linseed oil to keep down the dust. We always did that on Friday afternoon so that it would dry over the weekend. . . .

My first year of teaching was indeed a memorable year for me. Despite the challenges, my first school, Mitchell Run, is one that I re-member fondly. The physical evidence of any building has long since disappeared under the water of Taylorsville Lake. I learned so much there.

I am sure I made many mistakes but the experience started me on the road to a rewarding life of 34 years as an elementary teacher. When I refer to my former boys and girls, my family and friends remind me that they are now gray-haired and nearly as old as I am.

Hilda Snider, Taylorsville, "Hilda Snider Recalls Teaching at Mitchell Run," Reflections, *February 2006*

ONE-ROOM CAREER

I was attending a business college in Nashville, and on a visit home here in Wayne County, Superintendent Ira Bell saw me and told me he needed someone to finish teaching at Langham School, located in a remote section in Wayne County. The teacher had quit to take her regular high school position when high school began.

That was during the war years, and many male teachers were in military service. Also, many female teachers left for higher paying jobs in factories. I was very unqualified for this teaching job, but I accepted it.

That was back in very rough times, so I rode a U.S. Mail truck to the nearest post office, then walked about two miles to the schoolhouse along with fourteen pupils. The parents and pupils were nice, cooperative, etc. I had to board in a house there. . . .

After teaching for one year at Langham School I was placed in Sandy Valley School, a location that was better for me. It had all eight grades, but many of the pupils were irregular in attendance; I guess it was because they had to walk such a long distance. These pupils were behind in their learning, and some of them were fifteen years old but still in first grade. But these kids were well behaved and their parents were so nice and cooperative. They were just glad to have a school.

I was not well prepared to teach, but the superintendent was pleased and complimentary of my work. . . .

I also taught in a one-room school in Adair County, as my husband was from there and he was home from World War II. This school was large in number of students. However, the road to the school was a dirt road that was dusty in the summertime, but passable. It was opposite in the winter, and I had to walk much of the way to get there.

I enjoyed everything except the school building was used as a church every Monday and Thursday. It took such a long time to get things back to normal. The seats had to be rearranged, books and supplies had to be relocated, but the people that came to church were helpful and pleased with my being there as teacher.

The next year I asked for a change and started teaching at Fairview. The road conditions were the same as before, but the distance to school was much greater. School enrollment was fewer in number but these children really progressed in every area. All the parents and the school supervisor were pleased.

Gladys H. Roy, Columbia, January 12, 2009

School Days of Teacher and of Her Grandmother

In 1960 I taught my first school at Rudd School in Magoffin County. I had twenty-seven students in all eight grades. It was a wonderful experience. I taught what I could and with what I had, which was a limited number of books and a chalkboard painted on the wall.

The school was located on the side of a hill on the left-hand fork on Johnson Creek. I had to walk a mile and one-half each way to school, and the students from various parts of the community had to walk farther. The building was a clapboard one-room school with three tall windows on each side, a cloakroom, and a potbelly stove in the middle. The water was from a pump located in the schoolyard.

When everyone got to school they were tired, eager to get warmed by the fire in the winter, then sit down and work on their lessons. The days were full and we learned a great deal. Classes began at 8:00 in the morning, then at 10:00 we had fifteen minutes of recess, and from 12:00 till 1:00 p.m. we had a lunch hour. Then from 2:45 until 3:00 we had another fifteen minutes of recess, then another hour of classes. School was dismissed at 4:00.

Everyone was eager for recess; we played many different games, and there were no discipline problems. All the children carried their lunches, some in lard buckets, some in metal buckets such as the miners used, and some in a paper bag. But one or two didn't bring any lunch, and two or three of the kids went home for dinner.

We didn't have many maps in school, and most everybody in the community had a Sears, Roebuck or a Montgomery Ward catalog. We collected maps used for parcel post rates and put them on the wall. We learned our geography, and we learned it well.

From that one little school that year, three of the students I had became educators, one an attorney, one an accountant, and various other professions. I like to think I had a part in their success.

I taught school up until 1997, but I remember fondly that year in the one-room school with no discipline problems. Oh, a fight or a little quarrel would break out every once in a while, but I always took care of it by allowing the offenders to talk it out. . . .

In 1961 I taught at Ova School, located in the community of Cow Creek. From the home where I lived, I walked down the road one mile, up the hollow a mile, across the hill, down the other creek for approximately a mile and a half. That entire round trip was about five miles each way. But I was young and I was healthy, and I had a good group of students from the first through eighth grade.

Some of those students turned out to be fellow educators, and I still see them from time to time. They all look back with fondness at one of the best school years they ever had.

This was a school in a little better physical condition than the one at Rudd, where I had taught previously. It had two rooms, but only one teacher. The first four grades were in one room, the four upper grades were in the other. I would put assignments on the board, and the upper grades would work while I was working with the smaller children. They were very quiet when I went into the other room to teach. Some of the older girls that finished their lessons quickly were always glad to work with the younger children.

Supplies were limited, but we had a better variety of books than what we had in the other school. Everyone was expected to learn; everyone worked, and everyone did.

I would like to say that my students were all storytellers. It was my practice to have them do presentations, and stand up before the class and tell a story. Oh, what stories they told, and with such memory of all the little details. . . .

This is a story about my grandmother, the late Linda Arnett Howard. She taught school in Magoffin County in a very rural section near the headwaters of the Licking River around 1899 and 1900. The culture was very primitive. They had even less than I did when I was teaching in a one-room school. Some of the children had never seen flatware utensils to eat with. They used utensils whittled from wood. About once a month my grandmother would cook a big pot of soup beans on the potbelly stove. She would carry her own flatware from home, and have the children bring a plate in order to practice with flatware.

Years and years ago, I ran into an old man that had been an educator all his life, and he told me that one of the most precious things in his memory was when my grandmother taught him to eat with a fork, and how it was an asset to him.

My grandmother said that on the last day of this particular school she baked gingerbread and took it to school, [and] the boys dug a sassafras root and made tea, sweetened with molasses, in a lard can on top of the potbelly stove. They had a grand end-of-the-year party.

Betty Jo Arnett Lykins, Salyersville, February 1, 2009

EGGEN AND SALEM SCHOOLS

My first day at school was spent getting acquainted with the students, issuing free textbooks, and making schedules for the grades: two, three, fifth, sixth, seventh and eighth. At that time fifth and sixth grades, and seventh and eighth grades, were taught as one class. However, one year the fifth and seventh grades were taught as one class. The next year sixth and eighth grades were taught that way. Often a child would have to take the sixth and eighth grades before taking the fifth and seventh grades. However, I didn't seem to have any problems with that.

The children were all from low-income families, and they all seemed to want to learn. If I gave them homework to do, they always did it. Most of it was done at school while I was teaching other classes.

At Eggen I taught about nineteen students more or less. At that school, Brownie Goodin's little sister started to school, supposedly in the first grade. However, the superintendent said she couldn't come to school because she wasn't old enough. That suited me because I had one less class. . . .

From Harrison County my husband, William, and I moved back to Hardin County to his father's farm. He taught in Harrison County for one year prior to being drafted into military service during World War II. In Spencer County his parents had a tobacco crop for him to care for until the date he was called into service. After William left I continued to live in the house with two babies.

In the latter part of July 1945 I got a call from my mother, who told me that Superintendent G. C. Burkhead wanted to know if I would come home to teach at Salem. Miss Helen Patterson, my high school teacher, had started the school in July. It was getting time for the high school to start, and she would have to go there to teach. The last of August in 1945 I moved home where my mother could care for my children.

Salem School was much like Eggen, only I didn't have the opening of school to fool with. I used the same scheduling Miss Helen had used. The only thing I had to do was get acquainted with the children. They were nice and orderly, so I had no difficulty picking up where Miss Helen left off and going on. The children walked to school, but they didn't have as far to walk as the Eggen children.

On Halloween the windows in the boys' cloakroom were broken out. It was getting cooler in the season, so the windows had to be fixed. Clyde and Margaret Hunt had a big brother that passed the school every day in order to meet with the bus that hauled him to high school. He fixed the windows, and he fixed fires for me when the weather turned cold.

Eggen and Salem schools were closed the year after I taught at each of them. Eggen closed in 1943 and Salem closed in 1946. The children were sent to Rineyville, mostly because the men teachers who taught in the one-room schools had been inducted into military service during World War II. Teachers were very scarce.

Grace W. McGaughey, Lexington, January 29, 2009

The Way It Was

Back when I started teaching in one-room schools we didn't have electricity, so during the summer the windows and doors were left open all day. In the winter we had a potbelly stove in the middle of the room that burned coal. There was a well or a spring for fresh drinking water. Older students helped to bring in the water, as needed.

About 1934 the state started issuing free textbooks to all elementary students. At the beginning of school each year the teacher was responsible for going to the superintendent's office to pick up the books, along with a new water bucket, dipper, new erasers for the blackboard, as well as chalk and any other needed items at that school. A load of coal was delivered each fall of the year.

There was a health doctor and nurse that came to school and gave free vaccinations for typhoid and smallpox.

The Clinton County superintendent, Carvin Reneau, came every year and talked to the students. He usually gave each one a pencil. . . .

My first teaching job was at Willis Creek School, where I earned a salary of $112 per month. The school was about a mile off the main road, which was a rough, dirt road. There were about twenty-three students that year.

I lived in another area of the county and boarded with the Choate family. Mrs. Choate charged me $12 per month for board, and she fixed my lunch each day. Dad took me there on Monday and picked me up on Friday. I walked to school the rest of the week, and the students also walked. Most of them went barefooted, but they still played in the schoolyard during recess.

One day a little elderly lady came up to the door, and I asked her to come in. After we talked for awhile she asked me if I would read the Bible to her. And so I did.

I always kept a Bible in my desk. Later on I learned that she couldn't read, and I never forgot her. Later, when I thought about her, I got the idea to continue teaching. That way I could help children and other people learn to read.

Some people came to school one day and brought materials for a Bible school. We had two hours each day set aside for studying the Bible, reading, singing, and artworks. Every morning for our opening exercise we had reading, singing, and recitations.

We went to school everyday at 8:00 a.m. and stayed until 4:00 p.m. . . .

Teaching at Indian Creek School was [a later] assignment. It was the elementary school which I attended. The Wolf Creek Dam was being built at this time. Thus a lot of people had moved away due to being forced to sell their land to the government.

I walked over Grider Hill, and there was a creek on the other side. They had built a swinging bridge in order to cross the creek. Some of the people left cows and horses there. The horses would run like you see them out west on the ranches. It was kind of scary if they got close to you.

I had only six students at Indian Creek, so we had lots of time to do lessons. That was the last year for that school, due to the building of Wolf Creek Dam. We had only six months of school that year because everyone, and the schools, had to be out of there by December 31 that year. Someone had written up above the chalkboard, "Try, try again."

My mother, Oda Marcum Stearns, was a trustee at the school. My dad, John L. Stearns, and an uncle, Robert Lee Dickerson, came to the school and did janitorial work.

Kolema Stearns Davis, Taylorsville, February 6, 2009

THE RIGHT ROAD

Lower Elk School, where I first taught, was a rural school located at Knox Creek in Pike County near the Virginia border. I had to drive across a creek without a bridge in order to get to the school. If the water was up high, I walked through a railroad tunnel to reach the one-room school. There was only a one-lane dirt road and the students walked to school. A few years ago a bridge was constructed to better access the area.

The school had no running water and no electricity. I used only a candle on my desk on dark cloudy days. This was the last school in Pike

County to have no electricity. Our school facilities were very limited. We had the old-fashioned ink bottle desk, hectograph machine that consisted of a gelatin base for the stencil copy to do our duplicating. We also had the old-fashioned chalkboard and erasers.

I was responsible for my own janitorial duties. We had to build our own fires in an old-fashioned coal stove. I used a sawdust substance once a month to sweep the wood floors, and used an old-fashioned straw broom. We carried water from a hand-dug well, which a student would typically volunteer to assist. I locked and unlocked the school door morning and evening.

Since no lunch was prepared at the school, some students would bring only a small snack, which they ate fast. They were so eager to learn, they would beg me to give them math problems on the chalkboard during both lunch and recess. They also loved to have spelling contests during their free time.

The 1964–65 school year at Lower Elk gave me more experience and prepared me more for my next twenty-six years teaching than any student teaching, or college course, I ever received.

I often look back on my career and wonder if today's students would be willing to make the sacrifices that my students made in a one-room school in a rural area to obtain an education that is so important to get a young person started on the right road.

Stella K. Marcum, Pikeville, February 10, 2009

Teaching at Douglas and Sims Creek

Sixty-two years ago, in the fall of 1946, I obtained a very exciting assignment as my first teaching position. The Pike County school superintendent hired me to teach in a one-room school called Douglas. I was also very thankful to be receiving a monthly salary of about $105.

At age nineteen I had just graduated from high school in May (about two months before that) but had earned six hours of credit from Pikeville Junior College during the summer. Thus the Pike County Board of Education was able to issue me an emergency certificate. That was also the first year for Pike County to begin having a nine-month school term for elementary grades, beginning the latter part of July and ending in late March.

I bravely accepted the task of going to Shelby Creek, a community about twenty-three miles from my home, where Douglas School was located. Since neither my parents nor I owned a car, I would have to go there to both live and teach. I remember very well the day my brother took me in his truck to that strange community, but I found a place to board in a private home close to the school. Mr. and Mrs. Tackett were very friendly people and were willing to take me into their home. They said, "We have seven children, but you're welcome to board or live with us if you can endure our large family."

I was excited about having a large family, as my parents had six children. I gladly accepted their hospitality and was thankful to get a good safe place to stay for only a dollar a day.

The Douglas School was built to accommodate a mining community; therefore, it had three rooms. In the early 1930s it accommodated over a hundred students. But by the time I started teaching there were only sixteen students, who were in grades 1, 2, and 3. Children from grades 4 through 8 rode a school bus to a consolidated school in another community called Virgie.

We used only one room for class, saving the other two to play in because the school practically had no playground. It was up on a hill about five hundred feet above the road near some trees. The only view we got, except via the front door, was provided by the six big windows on one side of the building. All we saw were trees, a path around the hill, and a cemetery. You could not see anyone's house unless you looked out the front door.

My sixteen students would line up in an orderly manner when I rang the hand-held bell at 8:00 a.m. sharp. We began each morning by reciting the pledge of allegiance to the flag, singing, and the Lord's Prayer. We also had a Bible reading or story.

During the school day we had two recess periods in addition to lunch. Most of the children brought lunches in a brown poke or paper sack.

At the end of my first school year as a teacher, I was thoroughly pleased with my students' progress. . . .

From fall 1948 to spring 1951 I taught at my home school, Sims Creek, where I averaged thirty-five students per year. The school building was constructed in 1935 and had a potbelly stove for heat. It had seats for about thirty-five students, but the county provided more if needed. The student seats were the type that had a desk built behind the chair so that each one worked on the desk that was actually attached to the student's chair in front of them. The school also had a teacher's desk and chair, a built-in bookshelf, and a nice cloakroom for coats and caps. We had a special table that the first graders could sit around in chairs.

At the beginning of each year the teacher would receive one set of books per student, two erasers, a box of chalk, a broom, a coal bucket, a pencil sharpener, and a water bucket with dipper. We were not given any paper clips, thumbtacks, construction paper, workbooks, stapler, etc. This lack of adequate supplies hindered progress, so I often purchased supplies with my personal money. However, one main teaching essential was provided, and that was a nice chalkboard that went all the way across one end of the room.

When I presented each child with their book I required them to cover it with a brown paper bag known as a poke. In those days we had to be very conservative. I was required to cover my books when I was the student. Pike County did not furnish free textbooks until 1931; therefore, my parents had to buy their own, but several families were too poor to purchase books. My parents told me how children in their class that didn't have books would sit with another student, as most seats held two children. It was about 1947 before the county system was able to provide free textbooks to our high schools.

When I got to go to Pikeville to the board of education's central office, I would check out twenty-five library books per trip. I would take these to school where the students could check them out, take them home to read, etc. Then I would take that group of books back to the central office and exchange them for another group. While I was in the central office I discovered there were pre-primers on the shelf. There were about four books in a series and I checked out one of each. The names were *High on the Hill, Under the Sky, City Days and City Ways*, and another that I cannot recall. I got so excited about these pre-primers because the first one introduced about twelve new words, the next book about twenty words, and so forth, that I got the address off the back of the book and ordered eight of each.

I also bought with my personal money a box of flash cards with vocabulary words. I bought cards for all of the matching text in first, second, and third grades. Some parents were able to buy math and reading workbooks for their children that matched our text.

The school did not receive any individual cups for drinking. So I took a wooden pop case and painted it. Each child brought a drinking glass from home and put it in the pop case.

To teach at Sims Creek I walked about one mile each way. But I was able to stay at home and did not have to pay board. All of my students walked to school, some as far as a mile and one-half each way. School was never canceled because of the weather, as there was no telephone service or other effective means of contacting families.

In our community people did not say, "What time does school begin? or "What time does school dismiss?" Rather, they would ask, "What time do you take up books?" and "What time do you turn out?"

When I began class each morning I would call each grade to come up front to the recitation bench, a wooden bench about eight feet long, with a back similar to a picnic table. I started with the first graders and continued all through the seven grades. The students would bring their book and papers. Sometimes that was their homework, and we would discuss their assignments. Due to time constraints I was only able to have each grade ten or fifteen minutes at a time.

For lunch the students, except for two children who brought their own sack lunches, and I walked a short distance to a country store. There we would buy snacks and a soda pop for five cents each. Almost everyone would spend twenty-five cents and have it charged to their father's account. Remember, prices were cheap! I would talk with them, teaching them to always enter the store in an orderly manner. I kept a list in alphabetical order as to who got to be waited on first. If anyone did not wait their turn, they were punished. After everyone bought their snacks, we walked back to the school building to eat. Lunch break was an hour (from 12:00 noon to 1:00 p.m.), giving us time to eat and also have about thirty minutes to play.

The most difficult part of my job was trying to help each individual student. I taught seven grades and felt like I was not giving enough of my time and effort to *each* child. Most of the children's comprehension level was average, although I had a few slow learners. I would permit the older children to help the younger ones with their assignments. For example, one thing I did was to drill them on counting, the alphabet, and flash cards. Most of the time on Friday afternoon we did not have regular classes. Instead we would have a contest in math or spelling. We would also have singing, recitation of poems, and riddles.

I did not have any fights, but I remember two students who loved to argue during a softball game. The various games we played included baseball, tag, marbles, jump rope, fox and dog, ante over, hopscotch, farmer in the dale, last one out, pretty girls station, red rover, drop the handkerchief, and needle size.

During bad weather, especially the winter, we played games in the classroom. And yes, I played with my students. I would actually play with the younger children and supervise the older ones.

In an unrelated event, one boy broke his arm while he and another boy were wrestling. Needless to say, we all became very disturbed and sent for his mother to come immediately. One of the neighbors drove the mother and boy twenty-six miles to Pikeville where they were able to get medical help. The boy came back to school with a cast.

Let me also say that if a teacher became sick and needed a substitute, they would choose someone that had taught now and then in the past years. Before 1940 you could choose people that hadn't even graduated from high school.

Christine Thacker Justice, Mt. Sterling, February 18, 2009

Teaching in County Schools

My first school I taught was Brammer Hill, located in the eastern part of Wayne County, about fifteen miles from Monticello. My parents hired a relative with a truck to take me back there on a Sunday before opening of school on Monday.

For about five miles out the road, it was gravel. The rest of the way was big rocks and dirt. I went to my boarding place and stayed, unless I got a way back to Monticello on Friday afternoon.

I taught there in 1946–47. The school was small and had only sixteen students total in grades 1 through 8. The school year was extended to eight months that year. My first paycheck was $125! At that time I was known as an emergency teacher. Teachers with degrees chose the school they wanted. We had the option of going far out in the county or not. I wanted so much to be a teacher, so I went.

My second school was Mt. Hope, located in northwestern Wayne County very near the Cumberland River (now Lake Cumberland). Just across the river was Russell County. With the help of family I could stay at home. From one end of the gravel road I walked two more miles on a dirt road through the woods to the school.

Mt. Hope was a small school, grades one through seventh. At this school we had a pie supper with good success. It was a poor community, and the children really needed all the help they could get. Shades for the windows came first, then other necessities.

I taught for three years there, then taught in other country schools, which were Huffaker, Piney Woods, and Independence.

The most difficult discipline trouble we faced were fights on the road to and from school.

Norma (Stephenson) (Coffey) Bertram, Monticello, March 5, 2009

A CLEAR VISION

The first school I taught was Jennings Hollow School, located across the mountain from my home. The distance was approximately three miles and the road was a fairly good county road. I counted myself very fortunate to be located this well, as not all emergency teachers were located so well. I walked to school when the weather was good, but in bad weather my dad would drive me to school when he could arrange his schedule of getting to work.

The community served by the school consisted of hard-working farmers who wanted their children taught well. Most of the families counted it an honor for the teacher to come home with their children to spend the night, and they really treated you royally and served the best foods they had. It was wonderful to be treated so special and it gave me an increased desire to work even harder to teach their children.

The schoolhouse was well built, and it had a blackboard across the front wall, eight large windows on the sides, a large alcove on both sides of the front door which was a storage space for coats, boots, lunches, etc. One side was for the boys and the other side for the girls. There was not much opportunity for anyone to bother anyone else's belongings, because there was no need to be in the cloakrooms, and they were in view of the teacher at all times.

We had a very large, beautifully decorated blue and white water cooler which sat on a table in the back of the room. It held two water buckets of water. When water was brought from the spring it was deliciously cold, and when it was poured into the cooler it stayed cold. On the table by the water cooler sat each child's cup. To go to the spring and bring enough water to fill the cooler was a chore that the older girls chose to do.

When a student needed to be excused to go to the outhouse, he/she was supposed to leave by the door one of their books which had their name on it. Only one person at a time was to be excused. If he was gone long enough to be concerned about, another student could be sent after him.

That first school had twenty-four students evenly distributed throughout grades 1 through 7. In alternate years grades 7 and 8 would be taught. If you had a good-working group of seventh graders you could manage to incorporate a lot of eighth-grade work into their work during the last half of the year. The older students would work extra hard to finish their work so they could have time to help the younger children. They loved to be the "teacher's assistant," and their work was great help to the smaller children, too. This arrangement was actually a lifesaver for the teacher, as there was such a small amount of time for each class at best. . . .

The emergency teachers were visited very often by the superintendent or one of the other officials in the superintendent's office. Sometimes once a week we would have someone with us for half a day. They were there to determine what we needed help with, and help us by answering questions we might have, or just simply give us the benefit of their experience in teaching. I must admit I was terribly nervous at first, but as these visits progressed I learned so many useful things that caused me to actually look forward to them being there.

This, I assume, was my first step of a mature teacher who was seeing for the first time a clear vision of what a teacher really is, and what her job is.

Lucille Hoover Ringley, Monticello, March 24, 2009

Chapter 2

Teaching Methods and Philosophy

In the days before a college education was necessarily a prerequisite to teaching, those who entered the teaching profession had to chart their own pedagogical course. Few teachers interviewed for this collection spoke explicitly about why they chose to become teachers or expressed their "philosophy" of teaching, but their caring and their methods shine through in the stories below and throughout this book. Then, as now, good teachers were dedicated to the same goal: providing their students with the best possible educational experience. That they were successful is chronicled as well in this chapter, with some stories of former teachers honored years later by their students.

Greatest Calling

The main influence I had that caused me to become a teacher was my mother. She was a rural [one-room] teacher, and she thought the greatest calling that one could have was to be a teacher in public education. She taught only about three years, then married and started raising her family.

When I started teaching, the salary was about fifty-two dollars per month. Of course, that was just following the Great Depression years. That much money went much farther than it would today, as that was before we had a lot of inflation.

J. Robert Miller, Rock Bridge, September 18, 2008

Falling in Love with Teaching

I was going to college at the time, but I went with my husband the first day of school to help him enroll students for his first year of teaching.

I got the shock of my life for I had never seen anything like that. I was asking the students their mother's name and their father's name; when I asked this one little boy his father's name, he said, "Me growed from pumpkin seed; me don't have a daddy."

I thought, "This is ridiculous." Anyway, my husband told me to just write down "illegitimate." That's what I wrote on his card.

Every chance I'd get, I went with my husband out to his school because it was new; it was something different to me. I got to helping the children, and my husband just loved his job. All he had to work with was books, chalkboard, and chalk. He'd show me how to do certain things that he knew I didn't know, because he attended a one-room school. By helping him, I fell in love with what I was doing, so I changed my major to education.

Georgia Lloyd, Barbourville, November 21, 2008

It's All in a Name

When I was born in 1932, the custom was to drive and bring a doctor to deliver the baby at the house. My father's car wouldn't start because the temperature was below zero, and his battery was old. He walked around the hill to our neighbor's house. That neighbor was Johnson County's school superintendent, and a close family friend. His car was a newer model and had a newer battery, so it started and they drove to get the doctor.

When they returned to the house with the doctor, my dad and the superintendent went into the kitchen to have coffee. When the doctor delivered me he told my mother it was a girl, and she said, "Her dad will have to name her. Our agreement was if it was a girl, he would name it."

The doctor went to the kitchen to tell my dad, and he and the superintendent together decided that I should be named Garnet for my aunt who taught at a one-room school near our house and stayed with the family during the week. My middle name should be Gay, in honor of the home economics teacher at the high school. The superintendent stated, "These are my two best teachers in Johnson County and this baby just might grow up to be a teacher some day."

I could not tell this story for many years in fear of the political ramifications it could cause our friend. Our friend later became state superintendent of Kentucky. When I was a freshman at Berea College, he ran in the Republican primary for governor of Kentucky. However, he lost, and I was deeply saddened. Had he become governor I could have told people that the governor named me and diapered me many times.

Another reason I should become a teacher was that when I was getting ready to go to college, Dad's lecture to me was why I should major in elementary education. He said, "It's the only profession in which you can raise a family in eastern Kentucky and live. If, unfortunately, you should become a single parent, you won't have to pay a babysitter. You can take your children to school with you and be home to care for them on holidays and summers."

He then added, "The salary is more than a waitress or a store clerk could earn."

Garnet Gay Bailey Goble, Flat Gap, January 20, 2009

Decent Girls

My daddy thought that all decent girls ought to be teachers, so that's why I decided to become a teacher. I remember one of my sisters said she was going to be a beautician, but Daddy thought that was awful! [*Laughter*] Daddy was kind of old-timey, and he just thought that since a lot of his family members were teachers, that's what all his girls ought to be.

Virginia Janes, Edmonton, September 22, 2008

Three Generations of Teachers

My father, Dan Adkins, taught in an elementary school in Jonican, Kentucky, for a short time. He later became an electrician around the mines in eastern Kentucky.

Dad raised ten children, then later became a Primitive Baptist preacher until the day he died. He was a big influence on my becoming a teacher. He wanted me to stay home to help raise my brothers and sisters, since I was oldest of the ten children. When I graduated from high school I wanted to go to college to become a teacher, so I packed my suitcase and was headed out the door.

When Dad asked me where I was going, I explained to him I was serious about becoming a teacher, and I was going to Pikeville College to enroll. After that day Dad went to Pikeville College every month to pay my tuition until I graduated two years later.

The first year I taught Dad gave me his school bell, which was used by him to get his students to come back into the building from recess. I later had my name, along with the names of my dad and son, who also became a teacher for thirty-three years, engraved on the bell.

I cherish this bell very much to this day.

Emogene A. Browning, Louisville, January 23, 2009

Good at Her "Books"

Many experiences influence our lives and effect our decisions. I became a teacher, and here's the story behind it. When I was ten years old, due to my father's illness he could no longer do factory work in Ohio. He and my uncle bought a farm in northern Wayne County. The roads were muddy back then, no electricity, and water was carried from the spring.

I was sent to McClendon School and was already in fourth grade. Teachers thought I was ahead in my "books." At age twelve it was decided I was ready for high school. I went to Norwood, Ohio, to live with my sister, and she enrolled me in Latin, English, science, and math. . . . I struggled in school due to the teachers, so I decided to come to Somerset and stay with my grandmother to finish high school.

It was twenty-five miles from my home. I missed my home, so I'd get a ride home, usually in the back of a neighbor's truck on Saturday, and my mom would take me back to school. After graduation at age sixteen, I still wanted to be at home. . . .

Seven of us graduates from high school decided to go to school in Lexington while we worked at a job in Dayton, Ohio. When the opportunity [came] to attend a six weeks' teachers' training course, I felt it was the right opportunity. I liked to read, and always prized a clean sheet of paper and a sharp pencil.

I received a one-year contract in 1947 to teach in Wayne County at Ard School, which was located on a big ridge. The quickest way to get there from home was to go down a hill toward Cumberland River, cross Faubush Creek, then go up to Otha Ard's barn, where I stabled my horse and walked on to school. I was helped to get there by Mom, who cooked my breakfast, and Dad, who got my horse, Charlie, ready. That was not a drudgery, as I enjoyed riding.

Along the road one morning some boys hid in a ditch and jumped out trying to scare my horse. Thankfully, I was able to stay on the horse, thus did not land on the ground!

Betty Holmes McClendon, Nancy, January 26, 2009

The Right Choice

When I graduated from high school in May 1936, there were not many choices for Depression-era girls. Teaching and nursing were the most logical. I chose teaching because I had always liked school and respected my teachers. With acceptance into the NYA (National Youth Administration) program, and borrowing $150, I managed to pay the $50 per semester tuition, and $14 per month dorm fee, by waiting tables in the dorm dining room.

So I became a teacher and am pleased that I did.

Maurine Everley Grant, Owensboro, February 4, 2009

Career Delay

During World War II it was almost impossible to find enough teachers to keep all the schools in Wayne County open. Sometimes they would bring back old teachers who were retired or let the very young people teach, who were ill prepared for the work.

In 1946 our high school graduation class was given the announcement that if we had the plan to become a teacher, we could take a summer term extension class from one of the colleges in Kentucky, which would be taught in our area and that would prepare us to teach the following year in Wayne County.

Several of us went to the principal's office to sign up, and when it came my turn I was told to include my birthday, parents' names, address, etc., which I did and was told, "Sorry, you're not old enough." Actually, I was only seventeen years old, and my eighteenth birthday would be December 12.

That was such a disappointment, because all my friends were already eighteen years old. However, this turned out to be a blessing in disguise because I went on to college and got a whole year of work done, and was then allowed to teach the next year, 1947. The school year began in July and ended at the end of January.

Lucille Hoover Ringley, Monticello, March 24, 2009

Lifelong Dream

For as long as I can remember I wanted to be a teacher, perhaps because my dad was a teacher. School was always my favorite activity, and when school was not in session, my sister and I played "school." We lived in a sheltered world in the post-Depression era, so schooling was our joy.

In the fall of 1956 I began a teaching career that spanned thirty years. The first five of those years were in one-room schools in Carter County. My salary for the first year was $1,874 total. I had just received my temporary certificate and was anxious to begin the career I had always dreamed about.

Patricia Gibson, Greenup, April 11, 2009

Above and Beyond

When I taught at Bull Creek School, Letcher County, there were three girls in the eighth grade. They had been told that they must take a county examination and make a passing score before they could attend high school. They were very surprised and began to worry about it. All three of them were very intelligent, so they wanted to get prepared to take the test.

I met with them and their parents to discuss our strategy to achieve this goal. The parents gave their permission for the students to be tutored after school hours, and also go home with me at night for cram sessions when necessary.

The students and I settled into a routine as the semester progressed. We became like a normal school, and the students were very cooperative and excited to learn new things. They were proud of their work and took it home for their parents to see. Two of these young girls were very shy and timid. It took some time and loving attention to win their trust and confidence. One of them became fond of me and often wanted to go spend the night with me. She was from a large family and just wanted a lot of love. We spent one-on-one time doing her homework at night. She made great progress, and we both enjoyed time together. She was a very special girl and now has a successful life.

All three of those eighth-grade girls and I worked and worked some more. They were eager to learn everything. They were horrified to even think they could fail the exam and not get the eighth-grade diploma. They even thought they would be a disgrace to their family if they didn't get in high school.

The exam date finally arrived. The girls were anxious and nervous, and so was I. We knew we had prepared for the exam the best we could. I waited while they took the exam, and after a few hours it was over. We were all relieved when the results came, but opened the scores somewhat frantically. Shouts of great joy could be heard! All three of them made passing scores, thus were now officially high school students. That school year ended on a high note!

Teaching in this one-room school was a great learning experience for me. It is probably what inspired me to become a teacher and counselor.

Shelby Jean Caudill, Madisonville, September 25, 2009

Creative Teaching

One of my best memories of the will and incentive of a teacher to teach concerned a little girl. She was an only child who lived with her mother and elderly grandparents. This little girl had no small friends in the family and no small children living nearby. When she came to school she was very shy and didn't want to participate in any learning process.

In order to get her to do any writing at all, the teacher tried to get her to write her name, but she wouldn't even try. So the teacher began making letters and making a picture story about a certain letter. For example, her name was Audrey, so the teacher made an A and called it a tent. She then worked with Audrey until she could make an A. The teacher followed this with a U, which was a swing, and a [lowercase] D, which was a ball with the bat on the right side.

This went on until the child could write her name without realizing she could do it. That was the method the teacher used to let the little girl see that she could write. The teacher realized that Audrey was more socially deprived rather than just mentally slow.

Pauline Keene Looney, Pikeville, December 8, 2008

Teaching with Humor

One of the famous teachers I had as a teacher was the legendary Joe Harrison Carter, who was a career rural teacher. He drove an old Model A car, and would let the kids ride in it with him. They'd hang onto the fenders inside. He'd drive along by bushes and brush the kids with bushes and laugh.

I remember one thing that happened one time during the class. He was teaching a class in language and would paint across the word *ain't*. When he did this he'd say, "Now, class, you're not supposed to use the word *ain't*. Don't use *ain't*, 'cause it *'tain't* right." He would then repeat and say, "It *'tain't* right to use the word *ain't*." [*Laughter*]

I never forgot that. He had a way of making his point.

J. Robert Miller, Rock Bridge, September 18, 2008

Paddling for Literacy

I remember as a student at Moulton School when the teacher got the attention of a first grader who had already been there for three years. After she paddled this boy, he suddenly learned how to read.

Hale Murphy, Eddyville, December 31, 2008

Leadership

My first time to ever serve in a leadership role was when I was chosen to be leader of a rhythm band in this one-room school when I was a student. The teacher chose me because I could keep perfect time while playing a musical instrument. I still do that today while playing a mandolin.

I vividly remember my teacher that year, and feel that was my best year at school. In all honesty, little things make a big difference in a child's life.

Hale Murphy, Eddyville, December 31, 2008

Students Learned from Each Other

The most beneficial things students received from going to a one-room school included companionship of all the different grades together, and teaching them to respect the different ages of the students; and lessons taught, especially the sixth, seventh, and eighth. What they learned in the sixth grade helped them so very much in the seventh, etc. Each grade helped the students so very much with their intelligence

The friendship they had caused them to respect each other, so none of them thought they were better than the others.

I thought it was a shame when one-room schools were closed forever. Back then I think the students learned the basics more thorough than they do now.

Mayola Graves, Loretto, September 9, 2008

QUALITY OF ONE-ROOM SCHOOL SYSTEM

As I think back about my days of teaching in rural schools, one of the problems of the rural school was the teacher didn't have enough time to give personal attention to each individual student. To me, that was the main objection to the rural school. You had a number of kids in all eight grades, and you just didn't have enough time to give individual attention to students.

However, I think a plus of the rural schools was that they were high on the teaching of fundamentals. Reading, spelling, arithmetic emphasized the importance of these subjects. One of the extracurricular activities at school was on Friday afternoons we would cipher, do figures on the board, or we would do spelling matches. These spellings were either railroad spellings or what was called sit-down spellings. The students stood on opposite sides of the schoolroom in order to compete with one another. When a student on the opposite side spelled a word, the student on the opposite side had to spell a word that began with the last letter in the word the opposing student had spelled.

When they ciphered, the children would choose to do additions, subtraction, multiplication tables, and division. The student that finished first would be the winner, and the other one would sit down. Then another student would come up and challenge the winner. That was called ciphering.

J. Robert Miller, Rock Bridge, September 18, 2008

STUDENTS HELPING EACH OTHER

In the one-room schools the pretty good students would work with some of the other kids in the next grade. What I liked about the rural schools is that the children learned from other kids. They really did. I even let them work with other kids. When the younger kids were reciting during their sessions, the older kids heard what was being said; thus it was a constant review process.

Virginia Janes, Edmonton, September 22, 2008

EXCELLING WITHOUT PRESSURE

From my point of view there were advantages to one-room schools.

I personally used my advanced students as teacher's aides to mentor slower students. These students and the underclass students loved their relationships. I don't remember ever having more than five grades in a first grade through eighth grade school. . . .

Students in one-room schools were allowed to excel in any and all subjects without teacher pressure. The more intellectually advanced students did their grade work and listened to the next grade being taught; thus they could join in the process by answering questions for the next grade level. I had students who successfully completed two grades in one school year.

In those situations I was at liberty to double promote a student without consulting with any other school official. I would ask parents to have a conference. This procedure was usually following notes I had sent home by the student involved. The same procedure was used when I felt that a student needed to be retained in the same grade for a second year.

Garnet Gay Bailey Goble, Flat Gap, January 20, 2009

Teaching Certificates Unnecessary

All the early teachers that didn't have a teacher's certificate had to take a teacher's test. I think they went to the county seat to take that test, but I'm not sure. I had an uncle in Butler County that did that. His name was W. G. Woosley. I'm not sure that he even went to high school, but he did pass the test, then taught.

Those who never went to college had to take the teacher's examination every few years.

Marguerite Wilson, Leitchfield, October 1, 2008

Successful New Teacher

Up at Brush Creek where I was raised, we had two schools, Upper Little Brush and Lower Little Brush. Kids in Upper Little Brush ran four teachers off. They hit one female teacher on the ankle with a rock, and she left at lunch. The other teachers also left when the kids got on their nerves so badly.

A board member lived right out from school there, and we fox-hunted together and so on. He decided to go get a teacher who was one of the best in the county—and who weighed 250 to 300 pounds.

The board member took him up there, and this fellow had a

briefcase. He set it down, laid his paddle out there, then said, "Now, I've come here to stay. If anybody leaves, you'll be leaving. I know you have run three or four teachers off."

About that time, an old lady neighbor brought in a bundle of switches and put them in the corner, then said to him, "Now, there's more growing where those came from."

He said, "I'll handle it. Thank you for the bundle."

Well, that teacher handled everything just fine. One of those kids became a school superintendent, another became a rural electric co-op manager, one an electrician, another that worked for RECC [Rural Electric Cooperative Corporation] and formed a company there, and all kinds of good students came out of that school. They couldn't read a lick when he first got there, but he molded them. He'd go down through the aisle, and if they didn't have their lesson, he'd say, "Unhu, you've been p-l-a-y-i-n-g."

He really made those kids study. He taught them to read, write, and do math problems.

Pat McDonald, Barbourville, November 21, 2008

The A Starts Here

I have tried many different methods of teaching, and here is what I did. For the first ten years I changed my method every year while teaching ninth grade so that I could get more out of it. So one year I decided I'd do reverse psychology. The night I got the list of my students, I fixed my roll book, and the first day I met with them I took it to class and put As by every name. I took it to class and I turned the book around, then said, "I want you to line up orderly, walk by, and look at this book, and I want you to look at your grade."

So they did. They didn't know what was coming off. I said, "Now, every one of you have an A, and I want you to work real hard to try to keep it. What I'm going to do now is not give letter grades because I feel you might not like it." Then I made a bell curve and a chart I put on the wall that told what points were what. I said, "We do papers in here, and we are going to get points. So we are going to keep the points, and then they will be reflected as a letter grade from this chart right here."

So I let them know what the expectations were. I always let my class know. I said, "You want to come up to standard, and we want to keep this A as close as we can."

Well, my poor roll book was torn to smithereens by the time the school year was over. Every day they would come in and look at their grades, then some would say, "Look at your grades and look at mine; I'm outdoing you." There was a lot of competition in the room, like, "I'm not going to let her beat me, or him beat me."

Daphne H. Goodin, Barbourville, November 21, 2008

Teacher Had It All Sewn Up

I taught one year at Price's Creek, located next to Edmonton, in 1962. I had only eight students. All year long I was expecting a baby, and I was sent down there because it was supposed to be an easy school. It was located in a wonderful community.

We had time to get all our classes done. I didn't have all eight grades there, as we had only eight students. Some grades had two students. That was about the time the Barbie dolls came out. Of course I sewed, so I taught the little girls how to make Barbie dolls' clothes. Well, not many years ago I got a telephone call from one of those girls, who now works in a law office in Edmonton.

She said, "Mrs. Royse, do you remember teaching me how to sew when I was at Price's Creek?"

I said, "Well, I don't know. We did a lot of stuff, you know. Because we had a lot of time to do a lot of stuff."

She said, "Well, you taught me how to make Barbie doll clothes and how to sew. I raised a family, and I sewed and made their clothes, and I just wanted to let you know that you are the one who taught me to sew."

I thought that was so very sweet for her to say that.

She was up where we file our taxes, and I called up there one day. She had been up there getting her taxes done, and she wanted to send her greetings to me through our accountant.

Zona Royse, Columbia, October 4, 2008

Best Way to Teach

One thing I think I did differently from anything you may hear today, I did not use my smart students to help first and second graders. I used a third grader or a fourth grader to teach the younger kids their numbers. I was using a third grader who was having a lot of trouble in math to teach the first grade. I did that because the best way to learn is to *teach*.

The best way to lose a good student is to always have him able to do everything, and not have to work. I had this one girl in the third, fourth, and fifth grades, and I had her to write term papers, write music, play the piano, and sing according to notes, the way they went up and down.

I also had a German book for first and second graders to read, and I had her learning German. But I didn't have her teach the first or second grade because she was just always used to doing everybody else's work. Instead, I would have a person that was having trouble learning that 3 plus 5 equals 8, for instance.

I used concept teaching; thus I would have the first graders with pieces of coal, stones out of the yard, or I would have kindling, and then have them make me an eight by using so many pieces. In doing this they soon learned all these facts, and that I was not a rote teacher. I was not a rote teacher but a memorizing teacher.

Irma Gall, Barbourville, November 20, 2008

Daily Difficulties

The biggest problem I had each day was that I would run short of time, because by the time you'd take care of the little kids, and then get to the big ones in upper grades, you'd be running short of time.

I worked that out. Some days we'd have English, spelling, and everything. I worked things out so that I could utilize my time.

One of the big problems was getting beginners to talk. I had to get them up on a recitation bench and talk to them in order to get them to talk. I'd talk to a child about things he or she does at home.

I'd pat one of them on the shoulder and ask, "Do you have any dogs at home?"

They would grin and say, "Yes."

I'd say, "Well, what's their name?" and they'd tell me.

Then I'd say, "Well, what do you do with them?" That would get them to talking.

I'd go on to the next student and use that same procedure. After a few days, I'd have trouble with those beginners trying to get them not to talk so much.

What I just described was one of my best techniques, because those young kids were in a different atmosphere.

Noble H. Midkiff, Whitesville, December 1, 2008

STUDENTS HELPING STUDENTS

The most difficult time experienced by teachers was the first forty-five minutes of the day, because you had to tell each of the six grades what you wanted them to do for lessons, one by one.

I had some slow learners in the first and second grade, but I had some really bright students in the fifth and sixth grade. The latter would help the slow learners with their reading and math. By the middle of the year the slow learners could take a test with passing grades.

This method worked really well.

Michael M. Meredith, Bee Spring, December 7, 2008

INSPIRING TEACHER

Times have changed, but when I taught school, I dressed up every day like I dress up when I go to God's house. I think children react to the way people present themselves. I always loved my schoolkids, and I think they could sense it. I took them to the bathroom and washed them as needed, and I took them clothes. I always kept extra a little bag of clothes at school.

When I was at Jeff's Creek, my one-room school, which was seven or eight miles from my house and was across the mountain, that was the most exciting and rewarding thing I'd ever done. I couldn't wait to get home so I could fix dinner, then I would sit up until midnight making my letters and studying every class. I went through every lesson that a teacher should know in order to be ready to teach the next lesson.

I'd have a little period every morning, like thirty minutes, so I could go over things with the older ones that were working with the younger ones. I also made a schedule for everybody so that they got all their lessons every day. Then I'd talk to them about going on to high school, but nobody up here has ever gone to high school. I asked them why they didn't want to go, and they said, "We're afraid."

They were real backward children, and I said, "You're precious in God's sight and everybody else's. You deserve to do this. You've got choices to make in your life, and the choices you make makes your life whatever it is. Sometimes we make bad choices, but if we think about wanting to live good, we'll think more about making good choices." I went on to tell them, "If you will come to school, and if you don't have proper clothes to wear, call me before school starts and I will see that you get them. I don't have much money, but I'll get you what you need." I went on to say, "I will meet your bus when you get there and I will look at your schedule and take you to wherever you are supposed to go and show you the route."

I had three eighth graders and they said, "Okay." They came to school from there on out along with the rest of the children. I don't know of anyone from there on out that didn't go to high school, and they loved it. They drop by to see me every day and say, "I'm so glad you asked me to come to high school."

It was so rewarding, but the interesting part was that I had never just taught a child to read and just watch them grasp the words; within a week they could say their ABC's.

Two little boys were in the first grade, so I'd have to spend time with them because I had to get them to learn to read. I'd think that if they can't learn to read, I'm a failure. They've got to learn to read because that's the key to life. Well, those two boys could read anything by the time I left there.

Daphne H. Goodin, Barbourville, November 21, 2008

Honoring Teacher

I enjoyed my teaching years at McClendon, and the students seemed to really appreciate me. On June 9, 2007, these former students had a reunion in my honor. Since the school building no longer exists, the reunion was held in the home of one of my former students, Doris Decker Hubbard. All of them seemed appreciative of their experiences at school.

Betty Holmes McClendon, Nancy, December 16, 2008

All Worth the Effort

A young man I had in school came back here for his grandparent's funeral. His name is Tommy Ferguson. Diane was his older sister. She was in the fifth grade, and they were both very smart children.

I was at their grandmother's funeral, and Tommy had two grown boys with him. He said, "Boys, come here, I want you to meet a very special lady."

These two fine young men came up, and he introduced both of them. He said, "Boys, you've heard me tell the stories of me going to Hebron School. Well, Miss Emma was my first teacher. Even though she wasn't there very long, she taught some of the most basic, some of the most wonderful lessons that I have ever learned, and I can remember those lessons. She would read a Bible story every morning, and she would point out a moral, or principle, or a character-building trait that would help us through life. I must say that she gave me as good a foundation as I could have gotten anywhere."

I said, "Tommy, everything I've ever gone through, every trial—it was worth it for that one statement you just made. That's the reward of seeing your students do well."

He's head of a big corporation in Indiana.

Emma Walker, Eddyville, October 7, 2008

Appreciated Later

At the time I was teaching, sometimes the kids did not like me because I was strict, but since I retired I've had so many of my former students tell me how much they appreciated me.

I'm most proud of my career in how well my students were able to do in life. I can't think of anything that pleases me more than to hear of the success of my students. Those kids from Callebs Creek, when they see me they'll give me a hug, even now.

Joyce Campbell Buchanan, Barbourville, November 21, 2008

Inspiration

In July 2008 I went home to Spencer County to attend my sixtieth high school reunion. One of my former fifth-grade students had previously been in contact with me. My wife and I had lunch with him and his lovely wife. He had continued through college and eventually became a principal in the Jefferson County school system.

Even though I was in my teens when I taught him at Fairview School, he said that I had been an inspiration for him to continue in the field of education. He presented me with a beautiful painting of the old school, complete with the homemade flagpole.

Although my teaching career was cut short in order to attend the U.S. Naval Academy, that was a time in my life that I shall always remember and cherish. Today's students and many teachers take too much for granted.

William H. Nicholls Jr., The Villages, Fla., December 14, 2008

Chapter 3

BAD BOYS AND GIRLS

A recurring theme of the teachers whose stories grace this book is that they taught in a kinder, gentler era in which students respected their elders and misbehavior was limited to relatively harmless pranks and the occasional youthful defiance of authority, quite unlike the horrors that today's teachers often face. But even back then teachers sometimes encountered dangerous delinquents—and not all of them were students, as a few of the stories herein indicate.

ARSON AND FIREARMS

I typically didn't think we needed to spank, but one time this little twelve-year-old boy went out of the schoolroom through the only door we had. The schoolhouse was setting up about three wooden steps, and this boy set fire to the steps. After we got the fire out, I spanked that boy!

A week later he shot at me in the schoolhouse with a rifle and just missed me, but he didn't miss very far. Before he could straighten up and reload, I was right behind him. I picked him up by his spinderless [*sic*] pants and took him to his house, which was up the creek a little ways. I had a little talk with his daddy, so that was the last I had of that.

Irma Gall, Barbourville, November 20, 2008

VIOLENCE AT THE SWINGS

Something that comes to mind is about a bad experience. I had one child that lived in walking distance of the school, and she was supposed to have gone on home before the bus came by there to pick up the ones that were to be transported.

We were very fortunate to get a swing set, and this girl was swinging on the swing and one of the boys got aggravated at her for some reason. I never did find out what that problem was about.

Anyway, Brenda was swinging, and Dennis, whatever his problem was, took another swing and as Brenda started swinging toward him, he let that swing go and it hit her in the mouth. It cut her lips.

She came into the school crying and bleeding. It even broke two of her teeth. I never did find her teeth. I don't know whether she swallowed them or what. But we could not even find her teeth. I told her, "Brenda, you should have gone on home. If you would have gone on home like you were supposed to do, this would not have happened."

She had to go to the dentist after that and get two teeth capped in order to repair them.

Of course I lectured him, too, and I lectured the whole school the next morning when they were all together, telling them that they were not to do things like that. I said, "If anything like this happens again, I will have someone on the school board come out here to take those swings down, and you will not have a swing."

That settled it. I didn't have any more trouble about the swing.

Emma Walker, Eddyville, October 7, 2008

Bad Boy Turns Good

The year after my husband began teaching, Mr. Lay, the superintendent of Knox County schools, came to my daddy and said, "I've got a job for your daughter, but I'm not sure you'll want her to take it. It will be teaching a one-room school at Wilton. It had three teachers last year, but couldn't keep any of them. Your daughter is awful young, and I hate to put her out there, but I really need a teacher desperately. Your son-in-law has done a fine job, so I thought maybe your daughter would be interested."

Well, my husband knew the community, so he said, "No, you don't take it. It is dangerous out there."

I decided that I would take it because he told me not to. So I took it and the first two months at that school went really well. I was doing the same things I had done in helping my husband at his school the previous year. I began working with the children and finally got them in groups, found out who could read and who couldn't.

I'd make me some flash cards at night at home, and was really getting into my job because I loved it.

It was on a Friday afternoon that we played ball every day. They wanted to do that because they loved it. Most of the kids were older children, in third grade through the eighth, but there were two in first grade. When we played a ball game I was the umpire.

On one occasion I called "out" to this thirteen-year-old boy, but he got so desperately mad that he said, "I wasn't out!" I said, "I'm the umpire and you're out."

Well, I thought that was the end of it. We had the weekend, then I came back on Monday, and lo and behold, when I got there that morning, he had burned all the books. He took all the books, put them in the stove and burned them. I could hear him. He was up in the attic, and the kids all told me who did it. They told me his name and said, "He's up there in the attic right now. Do you want us to go up and get him?"

I said, "No. I'm going to dismiss school, and I'm going back to tell the superintendent."

I told the superintendent about the books being burned, and he said they would send new ones on Monday.

On Monday morning when I boarded the bus for school, the bus driver told me I shouldn't go to school that morning; then he said, "The boy you had trouble with is lying on the path to school with a gun." He also reported this to the sheriff and the superintendent.

That did not stop me from going to school. I told the bus driver I would just take a different path to school. I arrived at school and all the children told me about the gun. I went ahead with lessons as usual until I heard a commotion at the front of the building.

When I opened the door, the sheriff had taken the gun and arrested the boy. Before leaving, the sheriff told me the gun was not loaded. When I got back in town, the superintendent said that there would be a hearing and I would be expected to attend.

I went to the hearing, and the boy's mother was there and she was crying. Her husband was in the penitentiary because he had murdered somebody. That's why my husband didn't want me to go out there. Anyway, I felt so sorry for the boy's mother, and when I looked at her, she said, "Mrs. Lloyd, he's a good boy. He just got really mad."

The boy was crying, too. He hugged my neck. Anyway, we went ahead and had the hearing, and I knew the judge personally. He listened to it all, then said, "I've never done this before, but I'm going to do it this time. I'm going to leave it up to the teacher. She's got three choices:

we send him off, put him in the school for boys, bar him from school the rest of the year, or she can take him back and give him a second chance."

I looked back at him and thought, "I don't want to make this decision," but I did.

I went to him and said, "I'll take you back if you think you can act right from here on out."

He said, "I promise I will, and I'll build fires for you every morning."

Well, I took him back and he was a model student the rest of the year.

I didn't get to go back to that school the next year. Everything went fine after that and I had no problems.

Georgia Lloyd, Barbourville, November 21, 2008

Teacher Misbehaves

This friend of mine taught sixth grade. Students claimed that on one rainy day they couldn't go outside, and he [the teacher] was having them play blindfold inside. They blindfolded him and he went around and he touched her [one of the students], and another time he looked down her blouse. She went and told the principal, and they debated as what to do about it. They then told the superintendent.

The next year they didn't let him teach sixth grade. They assigned him to Moccasin, the only one-room school left in Metcalfe County. But he refused. He quit teaching, and wouldn't teach anymore.

It was a stupid thing letting them blindfold him and going around doing that. I think it may have been that some of the girls were kind of feisty, and they wanted to make a big to-do out of it. The girls claimed it happened, but it might not have. Of course, the principal got very upset when he heard about it. They then called the superintendent.

Billie Sue Blakeman, Edmonton, September 22, 2008

Dangerous Boy

[When I began teaching,] I was eighteen years old and had a sixteen-year-old boy who was in the eighth grade. He would scare small children with an open knife, and when I started to take the knife from him he would not give it to me, so I slapped him in the face.

He left school that day and did not return.

Myrle Dunning, Marion, December 23, 2008

Career Plans

After I taught at Norfork in Trimble County, I taught for one year in Indiana. I had the fourth grade and the fifth grade in an annex to the Gilford School in Lawrenceburg. The saddest thing that happened to me there was that one of the boys was definitely planning to be an outlaw. He was planning to be a gang leader, and he would say so. He would say that he would go into town at night and on weekends, and some of the boys would gather together.

He would say, "I'm going to be a gang leader when I grow up."

That was sad. I don't know what became of him.

Virginia DeBoe, Eddyville, October 7, 2008

Throwing Rocks

One of the boys at Station Camp there in Estill County came out right at school to visit for a minute. There was some sort of altercation over a cap or something. Well, this boy started throwing rocks at the school and was trying to get in. That was scary.

The father of the little boy that was throwing the rocks came and took his son away. I read in my father's diary something I had forgotten. He wrote that my mother had gone with me the next day to school, and that the boy was committed to Eastern State Hospital for mental reasons.

Maryanna Barnes, Frankfort, October 14, 2008

Bad Role Model

I won't call the name of this school, but one day a state trooper came to the door and asked to see one of my sixth-grade boys. It was a still that was involved, and this boy had been helping his dad produce moonshine whiskey.

I won't finish the story, but it was an interesting situation.

Maryanna Barnes, Frankfort, October 14, 2008

God Promotes Literacy

When I was teaching at the local elementary school, they grouped this room and put all slow-learning students in one class. There were twenty-three of them in eighth grade, most of whom couldn't read. They didn't want to learn to read.

They were in the eighth grade and couldn't read, and some of them couldn't sign their names. I said to one boy, "Son, at least you can learn to sign your name. If you don't learn, what are you going to do?"

He said, "When I'm sixteen, I'm going to quit school. I'll get me a draw, which means a welfare check, and set under that big oak tree and work on a '56 Chevrolet."

Well, that's what he did, but later on he became a preacher. I don't know whether God showed him how to read or what, but he went over here to Union College and took some classes in order to get a GED, and I reckon he is reading now.

Pat McDonald, Barbourville, November 21, 2008

Going Backward

One of the funny things that took place is that the administration came out and tested the students at the beginning of school, and they ranked fourth grade during the first month in eighth grade.

When school was about to be out, they came back to school and retested. This time they ranked third grade, eighth month. They had gone backward.

The administrators said, "Mr. McDonald, what are you doing here? They haven't advanced one bit. In fact, they've gone back."

I said, "Well, about middle of the year I decided to go back to zero and start all over with them."

But I was able to teach some of them to read a little. It was height and weight that allowed them to get promoted on to the next grade. Otherwise, they got too big for their seats. So I would write "Passed" or "Failed" on their grade cards, and I "passed" all of them.

Some of those kids didn't attend school on a daily basis, and you can't teach them if they're not there. Some of them missed twenty, thirty, or forty days. They just laid out. I told them, "If I could come up with a recipe to cure sorriness, I would be the top dog around." Some were just sorry and lazy, didn't have any pride. They didn't care. They went on to get a free check, and I had to work for mine.

Pat McDonald, Barbourville, November 21, 2008

Drinking and Guns Don't Mix

When I was teaching at Farmers School, we were in need of anything you could think of. All we had were the very basic things they gave us in the main office. So we were going to have a pie supper, but I didn't know all the things you were supposed to do to have a pie supper. I found out later that you were supposed to have the sheriff there, but I didn't know it then.

My parents were operating a store in Acton, Taylor County. They came out to the school and set up the concessions stand outside by the light of a lantern. There was a big crowd of people there. After the pie supper was over, there was a man in the neighborhood who was an alcoholic and would get kind of wild when he was drunk. So at the end of the box supper and most everybody had already gone, except my dad was still there. I was in my car and he was in his truck.

When we started to leave, this guy was across the road but he didn't say anything to us. We went on around him and left. Well, there was a family in the neighborhood that was really in bad financial condition. The children were actually hungry and needed clothes. They were still at the school. Well, this man that got drunk had a gun with him, so he shot the window lights out! Some of those poor little kids were still there, so they crawled under the desk, just scared to death.

That wound up going to court, and after it was all over somebody said, "Didn't you know you were supposed to have the sheriff there?"

I said, "I do now."

Betty Garner Williams, Campbellsville, December 11, 2008

Rated R

At Missouri Hollow School I had a really bad incident that happened with some adults on the playground when I had children in the classroom. That school was up in a hollow, and nobody was around. I had the forty-five kids in the room. We all heard this car drive into the playground. As you walked into the schoolhouse, you came into this little hallway after walking up three steps. Then you came on around where there were two cloakrooms on the sides, and that's where they put their lunches and all that kind of stuff.

When I heard this car pull into the playground, I went into the cloakroom to look out the window to see who it was. I didn't recognize the car or anything, but it just turned around and backed up until it backed the bumper up on the two bottom steps going up into the schoolhouse. I wondered what is the world is going on.

Well, this couple climbed out of the front of the car and got in the back seat. And there I was with the forty-five kids in the room, and you can imagine what was going on!

It was time for recess, so I thought what am I going to do? And the kids were wanting to go to the toilet, which was an outhouse. I couldn't let the kids go outside, because I knew what was going on. I kept thinking, what am I going to do?

I finally got my broom and walked over by the big boys and whispered, "I'm going outside to sweep out this hallway, and I'm going to ask these people to leave that are out here on the playground. And if I yell for you, you come, because I may need some help." I didn't know what I was going to be facing when I got out there.

I went out there and started sweeping that little hallway with my broom, and thought that they would surely wake up to the fact as to where they are, and what is going on, and that they'll get out of here. Well, I kept sweeping and swept right down to the top of their car, and they were still back there.

I took my broom and whammed the back end of his car trunk, and it whammed all over the place! The back door of the car opened, and he jumped out. There he stood with his boxer shorts and pants down below his knees. I said, "You get in that car and get out of here right this minute. I've got a full room of kids in this house."

I guess it scared him, and he was drunk. So, instead of going around and opening the front door of the car and getting into the front seat, he jumped back in the back seat and crawled over into the front seat, but then he took off! He took off so fast, he slung gravel everywhere. I never did see the woman.

Now, you talk about being frightened, I was scared to death. I guess he didn't know that was a school at that time because he was probably always drunk and used it as a parking place.

But what made all that so sad was that I knew the guy when he hopped out of that car.

Wanda Humble, Monticello, November 7, 2008

Chapter 4

VIGNETTES OF ONE-ROOM SCHOOLHOUSE LIFE

Perhaps one of the most valuable aspects of oral history is represented by the stories in this chapter: a sampling of sketches of life in Kentucky's one-room schoolhouses. Here the reader will find a mixed bag of anecdotes, variously humorous, poignant, frightening, and even tragic. Taken together, they provide a priceless portrait of the bulk of life—the unplanned part—in rural schools.

BARELY HEARD SCHOOL BELL

As a student in a one-room school, sometimes we would go out on a long distance from school [during recess]. At the end of recess the teacher would ring a bell, which was the signal for the students to come back in because it was time to start recitations.

One day we were out playing, and the teacher rang the bell. We all went in except one boy that didn't come back in. We were back in there for ten or fifteen minutes and he later came in. His name was Leonard Eaton. He was a friend of mine, and I think I was his idol. I was a little older than he was, but he liked to sit with me.

When he finally came back in the house, the teacher said, "Leonard, why are you late? Did you hear the bell?"

He said, "Yes, I heard it."

She said, "Well, why didn't you come on in when the bell rang?"

He said, "Well, the reason I didn't come in is because I just barely did hear it." [*Laughter*]

We all laughed at that, but that was his excuse for not coming in immediately.

J. Robert Miller, Rock Bridge, September 18, 2008

Educational Tangles

I remember these two girls that brought their crocheting to school. One time this boy got unruly, and Miss Gertie, the teacher, couldn't do a thing with him. So he set down between those two girls and got tangled up in their crocheting. What happened was he got wound up in their thread.

I don't know whether they did that on purpose, or whether they had their crocheting out there with their thread. They probably didn't aim for him to get tangled up in it.

The teacher got him out from between the girls, and set him down in another place, but I don't think she spanked him.

Blanche Demunbrun, Glasgow, September 30, 2008

Expensive Pie

I remember a joke on me as a student there at Merryville School. When Alma Miller was teaching, she had a pie supper. My friend William Denton Miller and I were small boys in about the fourth grade, I guess. We each decided we wanted to buy a pie at the pie supper. We each had a quarter in money; that's all we had. It seems like Frank Miller was the auctioneer, and he held up the pie. Somebody started the bidding at ten cents, then somebody bid fifteen, and the pie that William Denton Miller bought cost him twenty cents.

When they put up the next pie to sell, I thought that I'd bid on it. It started out ten cents. "Who'll give fifteen?" When somebody bid fifteen, Miller said, "Who'll give twenty?"

I yelled out, "Twenty!"

"We've got a twenty-cent bid, now who'll bid a quarter?"

And I said, "Quarter!" [*Laughter*]

Everybody laughed at me because I bid against myself! [*Laughter*] That was unusual, but it was all in fun.

That's an event that I remember very well.

J. Robert Miller, Rock Bridge, September 18, 2008

No Shots, Please

There were not a lot of events at school that brought in parents, but on shot days when the nurse would come to give medical shots, a lot of parents would come and sometimes bring their younger children to receive shots. I can even remember the mothers getting shots, but the dads didn't get them.

The little schoolkids would always cry before, during, and after receiving shots. They were scared to death of that nurse. Some of the kids would even want to run away from school while she was there.

I think the nurses expected that to happen.

Bige R. Warren, Barbourville, November 20, 2008

Taking One's Medicine

The county health nurse came to school to give shots to students. She was a very petite lady with red hair. No matter how big the boys and girls were, she managed to corral them and give them shots. One day she brought a German woman with her. We never had seen a German before. She was a really nice, big, tall lady, and she helped give shots. Even though we had trouble understanding her German accent, we grew to like her.

Those times when the students got shots to prevent infections were one of my scariest events. As teachers, we had to take our shots before starting to teach each year.

TB was a big disease up in this area. A lot of people had had it, and we were always told that if we went to someone's house, don't drink water there. That's why we were very careful at school so as to not pick that germ up.

Pat McDonald, Barbourville, November 21, 2008

Benefits of Unscreened Windows

When I was going to school at Merryville, located in Monroe County, the county nurse came once a year and gave typhoid shots. We were never sure when she was coming to do that. A lot of the kids were just scared to death by a shot. I remember one day when she appeared, this one boy, whose name was Leonard Eaton, was the largest boy in school.

He was frightened to death about taking a shot, so he was not going to get a shot! There were no screens on the windows, so he just jumped out the window in the back of the room. The school was located near the woods, so he took off through the woods and never came back to school that day.

He came back to school the next day, but he never got his typhoid shot.

There was a lot of crying by little kids at school when they got their shot, because it did sting.

Betty Jane (Miller) Pence, Franklin, Tenn., September 29, 2008

Avoidance Technique

At the Carver School the county would send nurses out to give shots to students. There was one girl, and every time she found out the nurses were coming she'd go to the outside toilet for girls, go inside and fasten the door from the inside.

She would stay in there until the nurses left. We really didn't miss her, I guess, but nobody else could go out there to the toilet because she kept the door locked.

Virginia Galloway, Merry Oaks, December 3, 2008

Mad Dogs

During my years at Jackson Elementary School we were advised to be on the lookout for "mad" rabid dogs. One day during recess someone started yelling, "Mad dog!"

Everybody started running inside the schoolhouse, and someone fell in the doorway. By the time I got there, a pile of bodies almost had the doorway blocked. I managed to make it inside without falling; then I ran and climbed up in the window for safety.

Laura Agnes Townsley Stacy, Barbourville, November 21, 2008

Fights

I recall students that got into arguments and fights at school. What they argued most about was either religion or politics. There were two different denominational religions, the Holiness or Free Pentecostal and Baptists. The girls would get to fussing over which church was best, and they get right into a fight over it. Most of the Holinesses wore long hair, and the Baptists always cut their hair. They would make fun of each other over their hair.

The boys would sometimes fight over little things. Maybe one would accidentally shove one down, and then the other would jump up and take his part.

Most of these fights of both genders would primarily be just wrestling with each other.

One time a bunch of us were coming home from school, and these two eighth-grade girls, Maggie and Mandy, got into a fight over something because when they got to the forks in the road, one went to the left and one went to the right. They had argued all the way to the forks of the road, and when they got to the forks of the road they started fighting. I looked around at them, and they had each other on the ground beating each other's brains out. That scared me so I started running toward the house.

I don't know what they ever did about that, but I think the teacher called them in the next day. I don't remember what punishment they got.

Laura Agnes Townsley Stacy, Barbourville, November 21, 2008

MORE FIGHTS

I never had any bad fights while teaching in a one-room school. I had worse fights by girls when I came to the city school to teach. On one occasion, when I was teaching seventh- and eighth-grade math, these girls got into a fight in my classroom and they really went after each other.

When they finally stopped fighting and left the room, I picked up some hair off the floor that they had pulled from each other's head.

Most of the other fights took place in high school, not in the classroom but out in the hall.

Joyce Campbell Buchanan, Barbourville, November 21, 2008

FIGHTING

I seldom ever had two students to get mad at each other and get into a fight. But it did happen some, and when it did I'd take them inside and talk to them. I'd let them go and wash, then sit right close to each other and have a little conversation so as to work out their problem themselves.

There wasn't very much fighting around a school unless they had an audience.

On occasion they did get into fights while playing games. When that happened, sometimes there would be injuries that happened.

Noble H. Midkiff, Whitesville, December 1, 2008

Aversion Therapy

During bad weather, the children at Eggen School had to have recess and lunchtime in the building. The floors were oiled to keep the dust down. A family had moved in during the school year, and they had four children. Their smallest boy, who was in third grade, wanted to wrestle with Charles DeSpain, which meant they would get down on the floor. Every day I would make them stop.

Being tired of telling them to stop, I said, "Alright, boys, my telling you to stop hasn't worked, so today go to it until you are tired." That's exactly what they did, and their clothes were an oily mess.

The next day the mother of the instigator stopped me and wanted to know what had happened. She was furious, but after she learned what happened I didn't have any more problems from her, nor her son. I told Superintendent G. C. Burkhead, and he said I did the right thing.

Grace W. McGaughey, Lexington, January 29, 2009

Mad over Marbles

Both boys and girls at Penick played horseshoe a lot. I guess the boys played it best, but the girls were also good. I also played with them, too. And we also used to play marbles, a game over which we had a lot of "rounds."

We'd make a circle and put marbles in it. The players would keep each marble they won, so we had a lot of rounds over that. One of the funniest things that happened dealt with one little Roach boy who was high-tempered. And the kids would aggravate him to make him mad. Then, he'd double up his fists and come after them like he was going to really fight.

The others would laugh at him when he did this, and that made him madder than ever. I don't think he ever hit any of the others, but if he did it was his brothers. They would also aggravate him. There were several of them in the family.

Virginia Janes, Edmonton, September 22, 2008

Bloody Nose

One of the worst things I remember taking place at White Oak was the time that Dallas Roosevelt threw the softball real hard and hit Clayton in the face and broke his nose. I remember that the ball hit him right in the face, and blood was pouring out of his nose.

Dallas said that he didn't intentionally mean to hit Clayton, but I don't know for sure. We were so scared, with his nose all crooked and blood gushing out, that Dallas ran all the way to his home to get on a mule and ride to Clayton's house about two miles away to tell his mama and daddy their son was hurt. When they got word, they came to school and got him, took him to the doctor, and then on to the hospital.

I don't think it was more than a day or two until he was back in school, but his nose was crooked.

I don't know whether Dallas did that on purpose or not, but I don't remember any of them getting into fights there at school. All the kids there seemed to be pretty good to each other.

Billie Sue Blakeman, Edmonton, September 22, 2008

RACIST EVENT

When I was teaching at Carver my students and I would go on little field trips through the Buck Creek area. There was a cave down there, and the kids walked into it.

One time there was a black man that lived down there who was a gardener who grew a lot of vegetables and sold some fruit. We went down by his place on a field trip to the caves and things.

On the way back to Carver a couple of little white boys in our group slipped out of line, then walked and did something to some of his vegetables, just tore them up or something. I didn't know about it until after they had done it, but when I found out about it I wrote the black man a note. When he got it he came up to school and talked to me about it. At first he was going to make their parents pay for it, but he didn't. Then he talked to the boys' parents and they got things straightened out.

After I found out what these boys did, I kept all students within the school building and talked to them, but didn't whip the two boys. However, perhaps I should have.

Virginia Galloway, Merry Oaks, December 3, 2008

BEFORE RACIAL INTEGRATION

When racial integration came along, there was a black couple that lived on the road down toward Coles Bend. I had hired this woman to do some housework for me while I was teaching down there.

She had a little boy, and she would bring him with her up to my house sometimes. He and my little boy, Charles, would play together. They were about the same age. I said to his mother one day, "He may be going to school to me next year."

She said, "Oh, no. They'd whip him and kill him if he went to school down there."

I said, "No, they wouldn't. I wouldn't let them. He's too sweet to be bothered, so he ought to go to school wherever he can."

Integration was never approved for that year, but he eventually went to a white school. His mother went to work for some family in Bowling Green, so they eventually moved down there.

Virginia Galloway, Merry Oaks, December 3, 2008

AFTER RACIAL INTEGRATION

The first black children I ever had in my class were at Red Cross after it was consolidated. After racial integration was approved, we got some black kids soon after that happened.

I'll always remember a little black girl that would come up and kiss me. She had the softest skin I ever felt, and was such a sweet girl.

She always remembered me after her school days. One time my husband and I went into a restaurant in Bowling Green to eat, and she recognized me. She said, "Oh, you used to be my teacher."

When racial integration began, white kids didn't treat the black kids like they should have, because I guess they got opinions at home that made them feel wrong. However, the black and white kids played together some. We had twin boys at Red Cross, and Taylor McCoy was principal at Austin-Tracy School, then came to Red Cross as principal. He worked so very much with these twin black boys to help them integrate.

Virginia Galloway, Merry Oaks, December 3, 2008

IMPROPER PEEING

My sister said that I told them [this story] and I believe her, but I don't remember this happening when I was a little girl in a one-room school. She claims that I had gone outside to get a bucket of water, and while I was out there and was coming back in, this little boy was peeing through a hole [in the wall of the school] and I dashed water on him!

I don't remember that happening, but she said that I told it. I don't even remember the boy's name.

Laura Agnes Townsley Stacy, Barbourville, November 21, 2008

Moonshine

This happened when I was going to school at Howard's Bottom. The boys and girls always played together, and the teacher didn't care. We'd always play cowboys, Indians, softball, ante over, and marbles.

There was a creek that ran down by the school, and one day the boys went off by themselves and wouldn't let the girls go with them. We didn't know why they wouldn't let us go play down there.

We found out one day that they had been going back through there for a couple of months. The teacher would say, "What are you all doing?"

They'd say, "We're just playing."

One boy that was in seventh or eighth grade had a picture of how to make a moonshine still. So, he had all the boys to bring corn, sugar, and everything to make moonshine whiskey. So they actually made it, then they all would drink some when it got ready. They all came back to school drunk, and some of them were as sick as dogs.

The teacher told some of the girls to get some of their daddies to come and get them and take them home to tell them [their parents] what had happened.

Boy, that was hush-hush there for awhile. They didn't expel that older boy, but he was the one that had the others to make whiskey.

Joyce Williams Ward, Campbellsville, December 11, 2008

Mistaken Identity

There were five families that walked down the same road that I did to go home. We also shared the same mailbox, and there was always a big session there at the mailbox every day to sort through the mail.

One day there was a little package in the mailbox, and it had chocolate in it. Well, the oldest girl decided to divide it among all of us, and that way we all got our little portion. I went home and told Mother and Daddy that we ate chocolate that came in the mail.

Well, they alarmed another family, then Daddy and this other man went up there and found the wrap peelings that we had thrown away.

Believe it or not, it was Ex-Lax! [*Laughter*]

And I think it affected us kids!

Duval Sidebottom Hay, Campbellsville, December 11, 2008

STUNG BY A JASPER

Another school incident occurred one day when waspers [wasps] had built nests near the ceiling of the room. As the room got warm, a boy near the stove jumped up from his seat, then continued jumping up and down to shake his pants leg.

Not knowing what was wrong, the teacher said, "Kermit, what is wrong with you?"

Kermit replied, "A jasper bit me." That was his slang word for wasper.

Pauline Keene Looney, Pikeville, December 8, 2008

DANGEROUS GAME

One of the playground games we did at this one-room school was try to find a yellow jackets' nest, then line up to see who could stomp on the nest for the longest amount of time. Each one of us wanted to be first so we wouldn't get stung as much.

Hale Murphy, Eddyville, December 31, 2008

YELLOW JACKETS REDUX

The sixth-grade boys at Farmers School discovered a yellow jackets' nest. They would not let it alone, so I kept saying, "Come away; leave it alone."

We were out in the woods in a very beautiful place having a really good time, but they kept aggravating the yellow jacket[s]. I'd say, "Come away, come away."

Those sixth-grade boys didn't always listen to me. So those yellow jackets swarmed and covered one of those boys. That scared me to death. If I had known then about stings what I know now, I would have really been scared.

That boy got white and he got sick, so I said, "I've got to take him home." However, I couldn't get the car going. We were sort of down in a valley or ravine, so I couldn't get the car down there. What I did was to enlist my seventh-grade girls to take care of the children while I took him home.

Betty Garner Williams, Campbellsville, December 11, 2008

After-School Snack

I remember that the schoolchildren passing my grandfather's farm on the way home from school in the afternoon would knock apples, pears, or other fruit from the trees. Grandfather wouldn't say anything to the children, but my grandmother would yell for them to get fruit from the ground first.

Throwing rocks at the fruit and knocking it from the trees seemed to be a skill. As the fruit fell, they would yell and the first child nearest would grab the apple or other fruit that fell to the ground, then run.

Pauline Keene Looney, Pikeville, December 8, 2008

And a Child Shall Lead Them

Dallas Wilson would preach every day while we ate lunch. He'd stand on a log and preach. He would preach the gospel in his own way of preaching. We'd all sit there and eat our lunch and listen, then we'd jump up and play ball. . . .

All grades of students at White Oak played softball, as they all really believed in ball games out there. One time we went to Penick School to play them. That was about three miles. A man in the community, Tom Shirley, had a big truck and he come and got us that day. We all got on the back end of his truck and rode to Penick and played ball. I can't remember the name of the teacher, but I remember she was an old maid. She stayed in a room-and-board house during the week.

After we played ball there at Penick, we had to walk all the way back home. I didn't know the way back, and Dallas Wilson had to lead us. I do remember that we all had to wade a creek to get across and go up a lot of hills.

Billie Sue Blakeman, Edmonton, September 22, 2008

CLASS COMEDIAN

I can remember so well when a boy didn't come to school one day, and we had this big tree right outside the school window. I looked out and saw him hanging upside down from a tree limb by his knees. He had a raccoon that he had tried to bring inside the school, but I wouldn't let him.

So, he went outside and was hanging upside down, looking at us from his knees, hanging on that tree. He was just hanging there upside down, thinking he was entertaining us with his raccoon! [*Laughter*]

Maryanna Barnes, Frankfort, October 14, 2008

CLASS ROOSTER

All the children at school were extremely quiet and tended to be a little standoffish, except one of the smallest boys who seemed to be always underfoot but never speaking. During my first week there, one morning the students were busy with their lessons and I was doing some kind of paperwork at the teacher's desk. Suddenly there was a disturbance that caught our attention.

The small boy was squatting on top of his desk, flapping his arms as if they were wings. A loud "Cock-a-doodle-doo!" poured forth from his upturned head and he proceeded to literally "fly" from his perch.

I stared openmouthed as he calmly sat back down in his seat and the other students went back to work without comment. One of the oldest girls approached my desk and whispered, "Don't pay no attention to him; he thinks he's a rooster!"

Norma Ramsey Eversole, Mt. Vernon, January 5, 2009

LOST PANTS

While teaching at Carver School, I sent three boys out to cut a Christmas tree. One of the boys was viewed by the other two as a teacher's pet, as they felt he got more attention than they did. So they decided to do something to him while they had him out with them. Believe it or not, they took his pants off and wouldn't give them back!

Many years later, one of my girl students back then told me that she remembered me lashing those boys really hard. [*Laughter*]

She didn't tell me what the girls did when the boys took off that boy's pants!

Virginia Galloway, Merry Oaks, December 3, 2008

Witness to a Devastating Flood

I attended Hurricane Grade School located at Fishtrap, Kentucky, Pike County, for grades 1 through 3. I finished fourth through eighth grades at Grapevine Grade School, Phyllis, Kentucky. I was in eighth grade the year of the 1957 flood that nearly destroyed the Fishtrap/Pikeville area.

I sat in a car across the road and watched four houses below mine float down the river. Our house was badly damaged, with the water completely covering the roof. It later required major repairs.

Stella K. Marcum, Pikeville, February 10, 2009

School Buildings and Farm Lost to Dam

When the Fishtrap Dam was built, our farm was taken from us, along with the local one-room schools. When that happened, I was transferred to Janison, Kentucky. I taught there for two or three years before that school was also closed because of the Fishtrap Dam.

Pauline Keene Looney, Pikeville, December 8, 2008

Fire Accident

This is a scary thing that happened at our school when I was a student. We had a long wood-burning stove that you poked wood into the end of it. One day we had salty peanuts in heavy cardboard containers, and they were round and tall.

Well, some of the boys had one of those, and they put some coal oil in a peanut container then put it on the stove. Somebody accidentally knocked it off the stove, and flames went everywhere. The fire got on one girl's clothes, and she got a third-degree burn and was physically down for a long time.

When that fire happened, I went out through the back window that was built pretty high up. I ran all the way to the high school bus garage and told some men that were working down there what had happened.

I don't remember just what they did to get the fire out, but they did.

That girl got a really, really bad burn, and I'm sure she still has some scars. Her legs and body were severely burned. There weren't many cars in the community at that time, so my dad took her to school every day in his car.

Betty Garner Williams, Campbellsville, December 11, 2008

Child on Fire

I remember that we had a potbelly stove at Laurel Hill that was used when a fire was needed to be made. The kids would get really close to it to keep warm. One little girl had gotten too close to it, and somebody yelled, "Miss Fitts, Coretta is on fire!"

So I leaped over a few desks and struck her down the back with my hands. She didn't have any clothes left on in the back. It burned her clothes, but didn't burn her. She spent the rest of the day with a coat on.

So I saved her life by jumping over those desks.

Velois S. Fitts, Winchester, as told to Deborah Evans Colburn,
March 17, 2009

Accidental Injury

Children have a lot of energy. They had to expend that energy one way or another. I remember one of the things that happened one time, and that was when some of the kids were pitching horseshoes. One of the little boys ran in front of the horseshoe stob and the boy that was pitching horseshoes hit him in the head.

His head bled rather freely, so one of the other kids took him out to Jack Wade's, and Mrs. Wade put some turpentine on a rag or something, and dressed his head. He got alright when she did that.

I'll never forget that because it was scary and frightening. But it truly was an accident. Those things did happen every now and then.

J. Robert Miller, Rock Bridge, September 18, 2008

A Lot of Blood

We played ante over, which was played by throwing the ball over the school building. There was a team on each side. When the ball was thrown over and somebody caught the ball on their side, they would start running around the building and see how many people they could touch with the ball. When they touched someone, that student had to move over to their side. The team that had the most players on their side when the game ended was the winner.

During one of these games, I had two boys that ran into each other while running really fast around the building. They knocked each other down, and probably hit something on the ground that cut their face. They were injured pretty badly. Back then the teacher was the doctor, the nurse, the mother, and whatever, in those one-room schools.

Fortunately, one of the boys was lucky because his dad lived down there close to his store. The father was running that country store back then. I sent a student down there to get his father. Dr. Stone, who lived in the Hydro community close by, made house calls, so he got him up there to take care of the boys.

He laid them down on one of the recitation benches in the front of the building where classes were taught. He doctored their wounds and everything turned out alright, although they did bleed quite a bit.

Virginia Galloway, Merry Oaks, December 3, 2008

School Is a Dangerous Place

One of the characteristics of the one-room schools was community quarrels, such as one family into it with another. Their kids would bring that problem to school and they'd pick at each other. If the teacher turned her/his head, these kids would have a little fight going on, like two little bainty roosters out there.

I'd go out and part them, tell them I was going to let them by this time, but to leave their problems at home. I'd go on to tell them we didn't have time for them to settle their problems here at school.

I never did have any really violent fights at school, thank goodness. But I heard that a lot of fighting took place while walking on their way home.

Most of these fights were about little picky things like "So-and-so said something about my sister, So-and-so said something about my brother," and things like that.

One thing that really tore me up was the time I heard one big squall outside, and I was on the other side of the schoolhouse. This boy had stepped on an old wire that they wrapped a broom with, and it had stuck right in the bottom of his foot real deep. You talk about a problem getting it out, getting him doctored and so on—that was hard.

The same guy in about a month or two was running barefoot through the schoolhouse, which was against the rules. As he ran, one of those big pine splinters from a plank in the floor went into his foot real deep. He was trying to get that big splinter removed, and it was attached to the floor.

He finally pulled it out, but it wasn't bleeding very much. Back then teachers didn't take students to doctors, so I didn't take him to one. But we did have a little first-aid kit and a knife. Their mom doctored them when they got home, usually by using turpentine and coal oil.

Pat McDonald, Barbourville, November 21, 2008

Severe Injury

Several kids from one family came to school at Dam 50 from their home on top of Cottonpatch. One of these girls came to school one cold winter morning with a towel over her face. She had put a can of potted meat in the oven to warm up so she could make sandwiches for the other kids. The can of potted meat had exploded in her face.

I had to get help from the men at the dam to get her to town to a doctor.

Myrle Dunning, Marion, December 23, 2008

Accident

On my first day of teaching at a one-room school, my dad took me and my books to the schoolhouse. The children were playing, and one little boy stepped on a broken fruit jar and sliced the whole bottom of his foot. That blood was just running everywhere, and I didn't know what to do, but he lived across the field from the school.

Well, I got him up on my back and carried him home. To get there I went down through the fields, and had to cross a rail fence, and all the other children were following behind me and stayed there until we got to his home.

His parents took him to the doctor after we got there.

Alma New, Monticello, November 7, 2008

Collision

The majority of the students walked to and from school. However, one or two large boys rode bikes to school part of the time. One day one of them was arriving along one side the school building, while on the other side of the building some small second-grade girls were running. The bike and the girls clashed at the corner because neither of them knew the other was coming. One of the girls got a one and one-half inch cut on the side of her face.

We were fortunate that a registered nurse lived in the community and could treat the cut and make a few beautiful little stitches in it. The cut healed up nicely.

Nothing happened from the incident because the rider on the bike was the uncle of the injured girl. However, we had several classes about playground safety versus bikes because of that happening.

Lucille Hoover Ringley, Monticello, March 24, 2009

Mysterious Overturning of Stove

One morning I came to school and the potbelly stove had fallen over in the middle of the floor. I figured the two boys that had come early to build the fire had pushed it over on purpose, but I couldn't accuse them because I didn't know for sure. The stove was not very stable, so I sent all the children home. I told them to come back on Monday, and that if there were a stove, we would stay. If not, I would send them home.

I set out for town, walking seven miles. I walked through fields, climbed fences, etc., in order to get home. Then I went to a neighbor's phone and paid for a long-distance call to the superintendent. It had been rumored in the community that the superintendent had said he wouldn't replace the stove when that one became unusable. When I called him he told me there would be a new stove at the school on Monday morning.

Two men showed up Monday morning with a new stove. They were dressed in their suits, white shirts, and ties. They asked me if some of the boys could bring the stove in. I said, "No, I'm afraid the boys might get hurt since they are too young."

You should have seen these two men's clothes once they had the stove up and going. The children went to the spring to get them some water so they could clean up.

Loella Lowery, as told to Jeannine Moore, Dawson Springs, January 10, 2009

Explosion

In 1948, eight years after I had been a janitor while a student, I was hired to teach in this same one-room school, Sims Creek, in Pike County. Now it was my responsibility to hire a janitor. I asked my twin brothers, Kermit and Kenneth, who were in the sixth grade, if they would like to be my janitors. Oh, yes, they gladly accepted. I promised to pay them fifteen cents a day to build a fire and sweep the classroom each day.

My brothers left home about 7:15 every morning and walked about a mile to the school building, where the first thing they did was prepare a potbelly stove for fire. They emptied all the cinders from the ash pan, got paper from the wastebasket, and placed it in the stove. Then they added corncobs and wood chips which they had carried from our house. I kept a jug of kerosene in the cloakroom to pour, just very little, on the wood before placing the coal. Finally, they added lumps of coal, and it was ready to ignite.

One very cold morning, my brothers were having trouble getting the fire to ignite properly. They had used matches, but the fire was just burning slowly. Palmer, their friend, had come to school early and volunteered by saying, "I'll get it burning." He then walked into the cloakroom and picked up a jug of gasoline. It was the wrong jug! Palmer knew I kept a jug of kerosene for my brothers to use, but he did not know there was also a nearly empty jug of gasoline. He dashed the gasoline on the slow fire. Boom! Off went the stovepipes. Blazes of fire shot out and soot went everywhere! The blazes were so hot that Palmer got his eyebrows singed. The boys realized they had an explosion, so they ran outside for safety where, by then, a few other students were arriving.

I tried to leave home every morning around 7:30 so I could get to school by 7:45, about fifteen minutes early. When I got in sight of the school building, I realized I could not see smoke coming from the chimney as usual. Then I noticed all my students were still outside. My brothers told me about the terrible explosion and that it blew the stovepipes off. Sure enough, as the students and I walked into the classroom, we saw the pipes on the floor and soot on everything. Even our books in the desk were a dirty mess.

I asked, "Do any of you recognize this jug that Palmer used?" I did not know there were two jugs in the cloakroom. Ricky, one of the fourth graders, admitted he had left a gasoline jug there yesterday. He had forgotten to take the jug home to his mother who needed the gasoline for her washing machine.

Our immediate need was to get the stovepipes back up quickly, as it was quite cold. I asked the students, "Do you know anyone we can get to fix our stovepipes?"

David spoke up. "Miss Thacker, my grandfather will come." I asked David and my brother to walk to his grandfather's home, instructing them to explain what happened and to tell Mr. Shelly that if he would come we would appreciate it. The boys did as I asked, but Mr. Shelly answered, "No." The disappointed boys came back and told us he refused. (I had been told that ever since 1934, Mr. Shelly was very selfish and would not lend any neighbor a helping hand. Now I know that rumor was true.)

We decided to make another attempt to get help. Kenneth went across the road to see one of our parents, Mr. Roy. He relayed the story to Roy about how our stovepipes were blown down because of the gasoline explosion. Mr. Roy came without any hesitation. He knew that his son, Dallas, and all the other students needed heat, especially on such a cold day. It only took Mr. Roy about an hour to fix the pipes. He helped the janitors, Kermit and Kenneth, build us another fire and stayed a few minutes afterward to be sure that everything was safe.

While we were waiting on the repairs, the students and I began cleaning. The books, floor, and everything else was covered with soot. We used old rags that I kept in a box in the cloakroom. The school building had no indoor plumbing, so we had to carry water in buckets from a drilled well. With a broom, cold water, and old rags, we tried to clean the room the best we could. About one and one-half hours later, everything was back in order and we resumed our daily class work, also feeling very thankful that the explosion had not been worse.

At 4:00 p.m., when school was dismissed, each of my students and I went home and told our families about the explosion. Our parents listened carefully to every detail about what we had endured that day. They, too, were very thankful that only one child was slightly injured, when it could have been much worse.

That has been over sixty years ago, but I will always remember that terrible morning we experienced an explosion at Sims Creek School.

Christine Thacker Justice, Mt. Sterling, February 18, 2009

Halloween Prank

When I got to school one Halloween morning, the neighbor's kids had the teacher's schoolhouse desk upon the chimney on top of the schoolhouse. Well, they had to do some climbing to get up there and put the desk on top of the chimney. They turned the outside privy, or restroom, upside down. We had to get some neighbors to set it back up just right.

These same three would also just throw paper and everything inside the school. So it took us about an hour to get the school clean enough so we could teach.

Helen Raby, Elizabethtown, January 10, 2009

No Smoking

We had to bring our own lunch to school each day, and every day at lunch time I'd have to look up at seventh grader Dallas Roosevelt Wilson and say, "Dallas, put that cigarette out. Put that cigarette out." He was smoking outside in the yard. Every time I'd see him he would be smoking.

He was so tall that I'd have to look up at him in order to tell him to put that cigarette out. He was tall built and a big guy.

I didn't see him in all these years until recently, but I went to school with his brother, Woodrow Wilson, who was county judge here in Metcalfe County for years and years. The last time I saw Dallas in years was at a funeral. I looked at him, and I couldn't believe it. I said, "Are you Dallas Roosevelt?"

He said, "Yeah."

He's a big man, and he now lives in Florence, Kentucky.

Billie Sue Blakeman, Edmonton, September 22, 2008

Smoke Breaks

I had one boy at Carver School that went to the outhouse and smoked all the time. Some of the other children always told me he was doing that. I got after him about that, and I think he still slipped around and did it quite a bit. He rolled his own cigarettes, using homegrown tobacco.

I spanked him several times for slipping out of the room to go smoke.

Virginia Galloway, Merry Oaks, December 3, 2008

Chewing Tobacco

I had a little second-grade boy at Antioch that chewed tobacco. He was raised by his grandparents who were really good people. This little boy had chewed tobacco so much that his front teeth had a little hole in them. He would spit and spit and spit little bites of tobacco out of his mouth onto the floor.

Of course, I tried to teach him about taking care of his body because God gave him a good body. I couldn't do much good with him about chewing tobacco, because he was going to do that regardless of whatever.

Helen Raby, Elizabethtown, January 10, 2009

LOSING LUNCH

When I was in a one-room school, there were fifty or sixty students or more in the classroom at Miller's Creek. The school sat between an old wagon road and the latest one-lane dirt road. The old road was on a hill back of the schoolhouse.

The boys liked to play cowboy on this old road, which was the same road we rode down the hill on while using cardboard boxes to ride on when the hill was covered with ice or snow.

The boys also began experimenting with chewing tobacco. A few of their parents grew their own tobacco for their own use. One of the boys decided that he would hold his tobacco in his mouth until the bell rang. At the last minute he would throw his tobacco away just before entering the school building.

The eighth-grade class was the first one called after lunch. The long class bench was near the stove. After this boy got hot he began to get sick since he hadn't had time to rinse his mouth after spitting out his tobacco. The longer he sat, the sicker he got. He whispered to one of the other boys that he was very sick. Before the other boy could respond, the tobacco-chewing boy ran to the nearest window, quickly opened the window and lost his lunch.

Pauline Keene Looney, Pikeville, December 8, 2008

NOT IN THE RULES

I'll never forget one day we were playing hide and seek. We had trees close to the schoolhouse. One little first-grade boy was hiding his eyes. I was standing close by and saw him peek and heard him say, "Boy, look at them run!"

Norma (Stephenson) (Coffey) Bertram, Monticello, March 5, 2009

Good Excuse

I was teaching at Kentucky Rock Asphalt Company School, and had a boy whose name was Wayne Ray. He would come to school dirty, and I would ask him why he came that way.

He said, "Miss Teacher, I didn't have any water at home."

So I told him that a branch of water was on his way to school, and he could wash there.

Then he said, "No, no, I can't do that because I almost drowned there one time."

Blanche Demunbrun, Glasgow, September 30, 2008

Loving Teacher

Ricky Doom thought "Miss Emma" was just "it." I don't know that it was in a flirty situation type thing, but every time I'd see his mother, she'd say, "All Ricky talks about is you!"

I remember her saying that. Ricky is a highway patrolman today.

Emma Walker, Eddyville, October 7, 2008

In Love with Teacher

There was a boy that graduated from the Montgomery School, and he was real smart. He asked me if he could come and take the eighth grade again because he wanted to learn a little bit more. I thought that was really good that he had that kind of attitude.

So he came back to school several weeks. He then asked, "Could I stay after school?"

I thought that maybe he needed help with math or something. He said, "Miss Helen, I'm in love with you and I just want to come back to school. It's too far to go to Auburn because it's almost three miles; we don't have any buses, and I'd just like to take the eighth grade over."

I said, "Don't you think I have a love affair? I'm not going to let you come back to school because that's not what we should do."

Shortly afterwards he died, and that was a sad occasion.

Helen Raby, Elizabethtown, January 10, 2009

Teacher-Student Romance

This is about a romantic type of thing that happened. Joe Harrison Carter was the teacher at the second school I attended. There was a big girl that would come to school. Her name was Mae Walden, daughter of Hezzie Walden, and she was Joe Harrison Carter's girlfriend. She later became his wife.

Gilbert Crabtree told me that, he being the biggest boy, that Joe Harrison would give him a nickel to take the rest of us out to play. When we'd go out to play, Joe Harrison gave long recesses. While we were playing on the outside, he and Mae would be courting in the house. They would get behind the door and court.

He was a lot older than Mae, but she later became Joe Harrison's wife. She was the mother of Bruce and Leslie Carter. Leslie later became a rural teacher, and a good teacher. Bruce became a dentist.

I remember that story and wanted to tell it.

J. Robert Miller, Rock Bridge, September 18, 2008

No Flirtations

I'm sure that the students had boyfriends and girlfriends, but I don't recall any stories about bad flirtatious events among the boys and girls. At least they never showed anything like that in my presence. They didn't even get together while eating lunch, as the boys all ate together, and the girls ate together.

Mayola Graves, Loretto, September 9, 2008

No Sex, Please; We're Students

When I taught at Big Creek the boys didn't have girlfriends up there. There were girls they could have had, but they wouldn't do it. The boys didn't think the girls were good enough for them. I do remember that there was a Richards girl, and her boyfriend was one of the Compton boys. They'd kind of get off and talk to one another and everything.

None of the students there certainly never had sex, and none of those students ever did act ugly, like touching each other and things like that.

Virginia Janes, Edmonton, September 22, 2008

Not Ready for Boys

I don't think I had any situations in which a boy and a girl were crazy about each other. Of course, they were still young and the girls were kind of "Humm," like they were thinking about that old boy, "Keep him away from me."

So I didn't have any students that were what you might say sweet on each other at that time. I think they were just a little bit too young for that.

Emma Walker, Eddyville, October 7, 2008

Stolen Kiss

One time I stepped out of the schoolhouse to talk to somebody, and when I came back in the girls were all upset. They said that one of the boys tried to kiss one of the girls. That was the closest thing to bad actions I ever experienced.

Irma Gall, Barbourville, November 20, 2008

Forbidden Kisses

Some of the kids kissed each other, but I told them I wouldn't allow that. When I caught them kissing, I'll tell them they had to quit that.

Most of that took place during recess when they'd go around the corner of the school and hide. You know, we hide when we do bad!

Helen Raby, Elizabethtown, January 10, 2009

Don't Kiss My Brother

The only thing I remember that has to do with kissing was when we were playing a ball game. We won that game, and that day at school all the cheerleaders went to this one little boy who was star of the game. All of them kissed him on the cheek, and his sister went up and spit on her hand and wiped away the kisses from his face!

I spanked her, but let me tell you that right now she is assistant superintendent of Knox County schools. She'll tell about that, too!

Georgia Lloyd, Barbourville, November 21, 2008

Spitballs, Not Love

My students were so young and diverse, I don't think the boys and girls ever really flirted with each other. But they did throw spitballs at each other and shoot rubber band stuff, but that was more or less just ways to tease each other. A spitball was something that they made by chewing up tablet leaves until they got really sticky and chalky. It would make a big paper wad that way, and when they threw it, it would splatter and stick on the person on whom they threw it. The boys did that to the girls, and the girls did it toward the boys.

When they did, that was usually why I would make them come up front in the room and make them look at the blackboard.

Betty Jane (Miller) Pence, Franklin, Tenn., September 28, 2008

Teacher's Mispronunciation

We were to have a Halloween party at school, but first had to clean up the building and wash the windows. The house was pretty, but during the Halloween program it was full of parents and visitors. So the room got kind of stuffy, and I said to one of the little boys that was in the back of the room, "Would you raise that window back there?"

He said, "Well, Miss Mamie, can't you say *winder?*" [*Laughter*]

Mamie Wright, Tompkinsville, October 16, 2008

The Silver War

I had one girl who was fixing the bulletin board when we were studying the Civil War. She just worked and worked, and I looked and she had written it as "Silver War."

We must have mispronounced it or something, so I said, "Take that down; we need to talk about how to spell it."

After we had a discussion about the correct spelling, she fixed it up!

Pat McDonald, Barbourville, November 21, 2008

All in a Day's Work

One time when I was on the way to Allens Creek School, Knox County, one family had five or six boys and they lived below the school. A lot of times they came running out to run to school with me. A lot of times I outran them so I could get the fire built.

One morning they came out and said, "Teacher, help us; something is wrong with Mommy. She is in the outhouse." That was very unusual, because there weren't very many outhouses in the area. She was having a baby. Well, I stopped and delivered the baby, got her fixed up okay, got her back in the bed. I then went to the neighbors' house and got a neighbor to come take care of her, then I went on to school and taught.

It was so very important to earn the respect of parents and their kids. The kids just loved their teachers.

Irma Gall, Barbourville, November 20, 2008

Teacher as Dentist

This is about me pulling teeth. I taught the little kids, and if anybody in the other rooms had a child whose tooth was just hanging, they'd send them to me so I could pull their tooth. Of course, I'd get toilet paper or Kleenex that I had there in the room to use in order to get hold of the tooth and pull it. I did that with my hands.

I twisted some teeth out, but if the tooth was too tight, I didn't do it. I'd say, "You've got to wait a little while, and then I'll do it next time."

One day I had a *fifth*-grade boy to come to me to pull his tooth! I said, "I can't get your tooth out." It was way back in his mouth.

I had this boy in the first grade to ask me one day, he asked me, "Miss Joyce, were you a dentist before you became a teacher?" [*Laughter*]

Joyce Williams Ward, Campbellsville, December 11, 2008

Miraculous Resurrection

This took place at Girdler Elementary School on Highway 11. My friend, who was my next-door teacher there, came in at recess and said, "Pat, I've got two kids missing."

I checked my roll right quick, and I also had two out. The teacher next door had two out, and the next teacher had three kids out.

We were located right on a busy road, and that worried us. We got to looking for them in a hurry. We looked and looked, but never did find them.

Finally, this one little ole boy came up and in a squeaky voice said, "Master McDonald, I know where they are, but you won't believe me."

I said, "Yes, I'll believe you."

He'd tell on anything and anybody. He was good at that. He said a lady told him where they were. He said, "They are up there in that graveyard covered up with leaves, playing dead."

That happened back when you could spank them with a paddle. So I got the principal and other teachers and we walked up to the top of the hill. I looked over in the leaves, and there the boys were, covered up. It looked like graves. The graveyard had a barbwire fence around it, so I stepped through that fence and said to the other teachers, "You fellows are fixing to witness a resurrection instantly."

About that time I hit the back of my shoe sole by popping it with that paddle. Those boys, resurrected from their leaf graves, came out running down that hill, and we were spanking them every other step.

After that, those boys never laid out of school anymore.

Pat McDonald, Barbourville, November 21, 2008

Touching Tribute

At Greensburg and Summersville elementary schools I taught fourth graders, and at Summersville I had one little girl that could do her math better if she could sit on my lap! Last Christmas she was at my house and said, "I want you all to take my picture sitting on Miss Duval's lap."

That was real sweet, and I have that picture.

Duval Sidebottom Hay, Campbellsville, December 11, 2008

Not Really Theft

The only thing I ever had stolen there at school was some new lipstick. I had it in my purse, and some of the little girls took the lipstick from my purse. They just used it, but didn't take it with them.

They didn't consider that as stealing. They were just little, and it was like what they'd get and use when they went to their grandma's house. They were just playing a sort of game, or when they'd see something at grandma's house that they wanted, they'd just get it and take it.

That's the way it was when I taught first grade all those years. They're really not thieves at that age.

Zona Royse, Columbia, October 4, 2008

CRIME DOES NOT PAY

Sometimes students did steal food from some of the others. One time, one boy got into another's kid's lunch box, and what he got was a piece of beef meat. As you know, beef smelled awful good when it was being cooked. But that piece of beef he took out of the other boy's lunch bucket was so tough he couldn't bite into it.

He stole the beef but couldn't eat it!

Mamie Wright, Tompkinsville, October 16, 2008

SINGING STUDENTS

We even sang gospel songs in our classroom. I had a girl in the seventh and eighth grade that was as smart as could be. Her parents did not allow her to go on to high school, and that absolutely broke my heart. She was almost my assistant teacher. She would stand in front of the classroom, and they would ask, "May we sing?"

She would lead the singing, and everybody knew the words to the songs. We would just sing, and have the best time. Right now, one of my favorite songs is one of the ones they sang all the time, "The King Is Coming." They also sang "Amazing Grace," "I'll Fly Away," and "How Beautiful Heaven Must Be."

I also read Bible stories in both the one-room and city schools.

Joyce Campbell Buchanan, Barbourville, November 21, 2008

NO PROMOTION, PLEASE

The third school at which I taught was Davis Bend. It was just wonderful, as I had the best relationship with students in my life. I could see those kids learning by leaps and bounds, and I was thrilled to death with what I was accomplishing, and loved every minute of it. And I thought, "My goodness, I get paid for this!"

On Friday afternoons I'd turn out school at 2:30 and we'd go three miles across the mountain to play a game of ball. I'd get home about 7:00 that night, and if we won the ball game, I'd take them out for ice cream. So I'd go pick them up that night and take them out.

I taught there two years, then Mr. Lay came and said, "I'm promoting you."

I said, "No, I don't want promotion. I want to stay where I am."

He said, "Georgia, this is with your husband, and it's a two-room school. The two of you can drive together, come home together, and work together. I may not have this to offer again."

I didn't want to take it, but I took it. When I went back and told the children that I wouldn't come back next year, we had the worst crying party you've ever seen. They didn't want me to leave. I didn't want to leave. After I left they called all summer long, "Please come back. Don't take that school."

That was so wonderful. I loved those kids. One of them turned sixty-five the other day, and I got her a purse. I even had their birthdays still written down.

Georgia Lloyd, Barbourville, November 21, 2008

School Shooting

I'll still never forget that kids of all ages use to make paper wads and then shoot them up onto the ceiling, and they would stick up there. I had to take a broom and sweep the paper wads off of the ceiling. The boys are the ones that did the blowing of most of the paper wads. It's not that the boys were better than the girls; it was just a custom for the boys to blow the paper wads.

I still have a big popgun that is real long that one of the boys used for his popgun. The popguns they used were made from reeds they grew on a stream close to the school.

They also had a slender piece of board wood that they'd jam paper wads into, then shoot the paper wads out, especially toward the girls. They also used dogwood berries to shoot toward the girls. Then, if a dogwood berry hit a girl, it really did hurt. Sometimes it would even injure the girl's eyes.

Mamie Wright, Tompkinsville, October 16, 2008

Putting Kids at Ease

Friday was a special day in my one-room school. After I noticed that certain families of children were eating lunch outside after it became colder weather, I asked the ones inside with me why the others didn't come inside after I insisted it was too cold to eat outside. The older girls said, "Mrs. Bailey, they bring biscuits with ham and baked sweet potatoes and they would be embarrassed." [If these items were all the children had, they would be considered markers of poverty.]

I went home and told my husband I needed to bake a can of biscuits one morning and fry sausage to make a sandwich to take to school. He agreed, and a few days later I took two biscuits with sausage inside them. At the morning's recess I made an effort to eat one biscuit and sausage sandwich, and be sure those boys were nearby and saw what I had. One boy asked if I had ever eaten ham and a biscuit. I said, "Yes, but that was when I was a child and my mom made homemade biscuits and put ham and jelly with butter in between them." I went on to explain that we took corn on the cob to school for lunch in August when I was young.

Beginning that day those boys began eating inside and asked me if I had ever eaten an Irish potato baked in the ashes under the fireplace or stove pan. I told them, "Yes, I have at a friend's house and enjoyed it."

The boys suggested that they could bring all of us a potato, and that they would bake them in the ash pan, and that all we needed were paper towels, butter, salt, and silverware. Each child brought silverware, and for many Fridays we had a hot baked potato for lunch.

Garnet Gay Bailey Goble, Flat Gap, January 20, 2009

BEET SANDWICH

When I taught at Antioch School, one little boy was named Buster. The students and I were always sharing what we had for dinner. Buster lived in my brother-in-law's tenant house and his family was so very poor.

One day Buster said, "Miss Helen, I've got something I know you'll enjoy."

I said, "What?"

He said, "A beet sandwich." What his mother had done was to cook beets and put them on a biscuit, a white biscuit. Of course, I didn't want to hurt his feelings so I said, "Well, let me put it in my lunch box and I'll eat it when I get home."

Believe it or not, I gave my chickens that sandwich!

Buster was a real sweet little boy. He was trying to show the love of sharing. The red beets had run all over the white biscuit. It almost made me vomit, but he would never know. He was a precious little boy I never forgot.

Helen Raby, Elizabethtown, January 10, 2009

Yen for Country Food

The kids ate lunch either on the inside or the outside of the building, depending on the weather. They had to wash their hands before eating, either by using a paper cup they made by hand, or by using a dipper to get the water that would then be poured on their hands. One person was in charge of dipping the water and pouring it onto the hands of the other students, and doing that was a great honor.

A food story that comes to mind happened at Ravenna, which is right out of Irvine. My husband's first cousin's wife didn't like her sixth-grade son going to Ravenna. I don't know why not, because it was a very fine school. Anyway, she got upset about something at Ravenna, so she asked me if I would pick her son up every morning and take him with me up to Pitts, a one-room school.

Can you imagine, wanting to send him from Ravenna, a really good school with really good teachers? Anyway, I took him to Pitts with me.

There was a restaurant right across the road from their house in the edge of Ravenna. It was a Wigwam Restaurant, and this boy's mother would send him over there to get his lunch every morning to take with him to Pitts School. Of course he got sandwiches and potato chips and stuff. But what he would do is take his lunch to Pitts and then trade it to those country children for biscuits and jam and stuff like that. He preferred that country food instead of restaurant food!

I think we finally told his mom what he was doing. [*Laughter*]

Maryanna Barnes, Frankfort, October 14, 2008

Miss Five-Eyed

Students fighting with students was the natural Sinking Creek way of settling arguments. They would either fight it out or run away. These things started when one of the kids said to another, "You do what I want you to do, or I'm going to knock your teeth out."

I came up with the words, "Okay, do it."

They'd look at me, then say, "What do you want me to do?"

I said, "You said you were going to knock his teeth out, so then do it, or else don't say it."

Then everybody would laugh! So, if I could stop it that way, that's what I did. That meant you had to have your ears open all the time. Kids were sure I had about five eyes! They used to call me "Five-eyed." That meant I had two eyes in front, two in back, and one on top. [*Laughter*]

Irma Gall, Barbourville, November 20, 2008

Boys Will Be Boys

My dad was also a teacher later on, but as a little boy he went to the same school I did at Little Brush. His brother went there also. When a water bucket got empty, one of them, or a friend, would go up there and rattle a dipper.

The teacher was busy, so Mac said, "I dare you to go up there and rattle it."

He went up there and rattled it, and that teacher came unwound. Grabbed him and wore him out.

My uncle looked out the window, and he didn't like school much anyway. There went a squirrel. He jumped out the window, took after that squirrel, and the teacher after him! The teacher yelled, "Get back in here! What's wrong with you?" . . .

Another little story comes to mind about the school there. These cattle were located around the schoolhouse. One day somebody got a piece of paper and slid it under one of these cow patties [manure] and took it up and put it in the teacher's chair.

Well, the teacher never did look down; he just said, "Good morning, children," then he set down right in the middle of that cow patty! It got all over him, and he had to walk about one-half mile to get cleaned up. He went on home and changed clothes.

These kids knew they would get him out of there. On his way back to school, he cut switches by the handfuls and used them generously. . . .

Then they put a terrapin in the teacher's desk drawer, and that thing used the bathroom in that drawer and scratched all over the teacher's record book and everything in there. You talk about a mess! Whew, whew.

All these things happened when my dad was attending a one-room school. He had some great stories he told.

Pat McDonald, Barbourville, November 21, 2009

The Yoke's on the Superintendent

One of the early Knox County School superintendents lived on the farm where I was later raised. He hooked himself in the yoke with an ox. He was trying to break this ox to work on the farm. He had a big field than ran all the way down to the church house, and that ox took off with him on the other side of that yoke.

He turned flip-flops all the way down through there to the fence. The fellows who were working there in the field ran over to him, thinking his neck was broken. He said to them, "Boys, unyoke the ox. I'll stand." [*Laughter*]

See, he made superintendent!

Pat McDonald, Barbourville, November 21, 2008

Buggers

My four older sisters were teachers. One of them was teaching in a one-room school called Palmyra. She came home one Friday and mentioned that her head was itching. On examination, her beautiful black hair was found to be infested with lice. She cried and cried and said that she would never go back to school.

Mother called them buggers, not lice, and she had two old-fashioned remedies to get rid of them. One was a concoction she called "red percipity," and the other was kerosene. I don't know which she used, but I do know my sister went back to school on Monday. She had a very tender scalp, but not a bugger anywhere.

She also received a warning from my mother to be careful where she poked her head.

Vera Virgin, Greenup, January 21, 2009

Itch and Lice

Have you ever had itch? I got a case at school. This family of five kids all had it. I went home on Friday, and my dad went to the drugstore to purchase some Red Pacific, and it did the job.

On another occasion I could feel something crawling on me and I had nats [young lice] all over my head. We drowned them by greasing my hair with fried meat grease.

Some of those home remedies really worked, and I survived that disaster.

Helen Raby, Elizabethtown, January 10, 2009

CLOSE QUARTERS

I left White Oak because the superintendent told me they were moving me to Edmonton to put me in the sixth grade. I don't know why they moved me, but they did and I was glad, because I could walk to school. I lived on the courthouse square and could walk to school.

The next year I was assigned to teach first grade, and they put me in a little tiny basement room that today would be just about the size of a closet. I had forty little kids in this awful little basement. They crammed us in there, and we had to almost crawl over one another. The water run down the walls in the basement, and the kids' coats had to hang onto the back of a chair. Every week at a teachers' meeting I'd ask if they would please have the agriculture boys to please build a coatrack.

Of course they never would do it. The kids' coats would hang on the back of a chair and get wet.

There were forty of us crammed into that room. A room like that wouldn't be allowed today, of course.

I don't remember ever spanking anybody out at White Oak. I spanked a lot of students later on, but not at White Oak. They were all good little kids, brothers and sisters, and kinfolks.

Billie Sue Blakeman, Edmonton, September 22, 2008

CHEESE WILL BIND YOU

Even in second grade, after a spelling class, I'd have them write sentences with the words they had learned. It was sort of going on a little bit with their own work, instead of listening to somebody else there in the room.

One of the smartest little girls I ever taught had the word "bind" in her spelling. She wrote, "Cheese will bind me." [*Laughter*]

She was a beautiful little girl. Her mother had been talking to her some about what foods to eat. So, she learned that cheese would "bind" her.

That little girl went on and became a teacher.

Marguerite Wilson, Leitchfield, October 1, 2008

CONVERGING PUDDLES

These two little girls, Nona and Cora Jane, would not use the restroom.

I guess they were afraid to use it. Everyday after lunch I would stand in the hall because the boys would squirt water on each other. The girls went downstairs. So I'd alternate; part of the time up here with the boys, and part of the time down with the girls.

We'd come back upstairs and have them lay their heads over and rest a few minutes. They'd start hollering, "Miss Billie Sue, Nona is pis——g." They'd start moving their chair back so they wouldn't have their feet in that stuff; then they'd say, "Cora Jane is, too."

They both did that every day after lunch. One would do it, then the other one would. Their two puddles of water joined, then got bigger and bigger. I'd push the buzzer and tell them that heard it to send the janitor with a mop. Well, before he got there, the puddles would join, and everybody is moving their chair back. Their puddles would go almost to the door. I thought, boy that floor is uneven! They were over next to the windows, and the two puddles would join every day and go across the floor to the door.

Those two girls would do that every day after I took them to the restroom. I decided that they were afraid of the commode. Anyway, the janitor had to come every day to clean the mess up.

I took the girls downstairs and tried to show them how to sit down and how to flush. I said, "It won't hurt you, you've got to do this and stop using the floor."

They did that I don't know how many times. The other kids would holler to tell others what they were doing right there on the floor. Of course, first graders would tell you what was going on! [*Laughter*] They'd tell you everything.

Billie Sue Blakeman, Edmonton, September 22, 2008

Death Wish

After teaching in a one-room school, I began teaching in a two-room school. I was telling the students that they would have to have some homework to take home with them. One little boy said to another little boy, "Have you got your homework ready to take home with you?"

The other boy said, "No, I'm not going to take it. Maybe she'll die before tomorrow." [*Laughter*]

Blanche Demunbrun, Glasgow, September 30, 2008

TREE FELL ON SCHOOLHOUSE

My granddaughter was in a college class at Glasgow, and while there she wrote an article called "Timber at Carver School." It was written to describe the first time I was teaching first, second, and third grades there. We ran out of wood and couldn't get any, so the teachers in upper grades called in, but the main office couldn't get out there to get us any. Then the teacher told some older boys to cut down a tree or two on the school ground, and then cut them up into wood. Truth of the matter is, these boys didn't know how to fall a tree, so the tree fell on the roof of the room in which I was teaching.

The tree didn't hit right on the roof's center where the rest of the children were located, but just a little on the back side. None of us were injured, but it scared us all to death.

I told that story to my granddaughter, and she wrote it up and it was published in her teacher's book.

Virginia Galloway, Merry Oaks, December 3, 2008

FULL DAY'S WORK

Some of the previous teachers only kept the students until noon. They let the kids go home at noon because they did not want to have them a full day.

One of the parents said to me, "Miss Fitts, you make it hard on yourself. You don't have to keep these kids all day."

I told them, "I'm paid to stay all day." [*Laughter*]

So, no matter, I was paid to stay all day, and that's what I did.

Velois S. Fitts, Winchester, as told to Deborah Evans Colburn,
March 17, 2009

PRETTY TEACHER WITH MUMPS

On the last day of school at Goff I had mumps. So I just handed out the grade cards to the students through the car window. . . .

This is about one of my first boys in eighth grade who recently gave Leitchfield schools fifty thousand dollars for a greenhouse. And he has told me that he thought I was pretty. He was about fourteen years old then.

We have visited some in the last several years, and that's when he told me that!

Marguerite Wilson, Leitchfield, October 1, 2008

Sharing

I was teaching reading at the table when a little boy named Harvey Junior looked at me and said, "Boy, you sure have big ti——s."

I had taken my jacket off because the blower was blowing heat on me and it was so hot. When he said that, of course I was shocked. When he said that, I said, "Let's go to the next page."

This little boy had never been anywhere and was very backward. I had a sharing period the last hour of school every Friday. The children could tell a story, nursery rhyme, sing a song, and anything else they wanted to share. I did this to get the shy ones to talk. Harvey had never shared anything with us. After a few months, one day Harvey raised his hand to share something with us, and I was so happy. This is what Harvey shared:

"Bill, Bill, lives on a hill, and he wipes his a—— with a five-dollar bill."

I was really shocked, so I looked at the other kids to see their reactions. They had their hands over their mouth, and their eyes real big. I said, "Harvey, who taught you that?"

He said, "Mama," then he looked so happy because he had finally shared with us.

What could I say? Harvey had finally shared!

Billie Sue Blakeman, Edmonton, September 22, 2008

Jimdog

I always took one of my girl students and her big brother home after school was over for the day. One day when we got there their little brother was there. Their mother said, "Come in a minute, Miss Lloyd, Johnny has something he wants to tell you."

Johnny said, "We got a mule today, and do you know what, he's got a jimdog that long!" holding his hands about fifteen inches apart.

He was talking about a penis! He called it a jimdog.

We nicknamed Johnny as Jimdog, and to this day I still call him Jimdog!

Georgia Lloyd, Barbourville, November 21, 2008

TEACHING IN A TENT

The second time I taught at Walnut Grove, which was in the 1940s, a windstorm had blown the school off its foundation prior to the beginning of the school session, and I taught in a tent for six weeks while the school was being repaired.

Bernice Shartzer, Caneyville, October 1, 2008

HARD NAME

We didn't do manuscript writing/printing like they do at schools now. We just started out using cursive longhand, and I wrote their names on the board for them to copy. My little sister was a student of mine back then, and her name was Jacqueline. I spelled out her whole name on the board, and then she said, "Sissy, what made you give me a harder name than anybody else?"

Because I wrote everybody's names on the board, my sister thought I had given her the hardest name to spell! [*Laughter*]

Later Jacqueline had a granddaughter, and she spelled her name Jaclyn.

Bernice Shartzer, Caneyville, October 1, 2008

GREAT BALLS OF FIRE

I think the funniest thing that ever happened while I was teaching in a one-room school took place at Bryant School. There was this boy whose name is Eugene Campbell, and he's a bus driver here now. He always comes to our reunions, and is one of my favorite students.

They called him Eight Ball at school, and back then there was the popular song "Great Balls of Fire." One time during recess—and sometimes I had classes during recess because our school day was longer, starting at 8:00 and continued until 4:00—I was in the building with some students, and another child came running in and hollered, "Great balls of fire!" and I thought he said, "Eight Ball's on fire!"

That is the thing we tell when we have reunions.

Zona Royse, Columbia, October 4, 2008

Killer Student

One day I was trying to show off at school, and we studied Alexander Hamilton and Aaron Burr. We were role-playing and this one kid was pretending to be Alexander Hamilton. So when the supervising teacher came in, I was going to show off. Then I asked the students, "Okay, who killed Aaron Burr?"

A big smile came on this boy's face, and his big brown eyes beamed as he said, "I did!" He remembered his part!

Maryanna Barnes, Frankfort, October 14, 2008

Airplane Coming!

When I was teaching school at Hamilton, that was in the early days of the airplane. When an airplane was coming in our direction, we could hear it and all the kids would become alert and straighten up.

I would dismiss classes until that airplane went over.

Mamie Wright, Tompkinsville, October 16, 2008

Students Cared for Teacher's Baby

When I was teaching at Forest Grove, and had been for four years, they called me and told me this was going to be the last year for Forest Grove, and wanted me to go back out there and teach.

I said to the superintendent, "I can't, Mrs. Burris. I've got this baby and I don't have anybody to keep him."

She said, "You won't have but about fourteen children. Just take the baby with you."

Well, I took my baby with me, and the children just fell in love with him and took care of him all the time.

Duval Sidebottom Hay, Campbellsville, December 11, 2008

Lunch Lion

At the time I was teaching my first school at Farmers here in Taylor County, the school building was kind of up in the hills and wasn't very far from Casey County, where you really got into some hills. I would come back down to where my dad ran a grocery story, and the men there would always laugh at me at things I would tell. They would make fun of me and say I was too little to teach school.

I had this little '44 coupe car, my first car that I drove. One morning I pulled up into the schoolyard, and those children just descended on me from every side, yelling, "Miss Garner, Miss Garner, come see these tracks; there's been a lion here!"

I said, "Oh, it's a big dog, not a lion."

Of course we took our lunch, and when we'd eat our lunch we'd sit out under a tree and throw scraps of food onto the ground.

Well, when I saw the footprints, I decided it was a big lion, too! So I'd go back down to the country store and tell what I saw to people sitting around the stove. They just made fun of me and laughed about me seeing a mountain lion.

Well, it wasn't but just a few days until a mountain lion was killed on up in Casey County in the hills. So we had had a mountain lion that had been eating our scraps of food from our lunch buckets.

Betty Garner Williams, Campbellsville, December 11, 2008

Fetching Water . . . Eventually

One little boy was tired and bored and couldn't do much work. So I asked Buford if he would like to go to the spring. He left as he said, "Yes, I would love to go."

So he left and was gone a little while, then came back and stuck his head right around the door and said, "Miss Duval, do you want me to take the bucket?" [*Laughter*]

I said, "Yes, yes."

He was gone a little while, then came back and said, "Miss Duval, do you want me to get the bucket full?"

Duval Sidebottom Hay, Campbellsville, December 11, 2008

Don't Forget the Clorox

I will never forget . . . when our visiting nurse, Miss Lula Johnson, came to our school. She was a wonderful, caring person. On this particular day while she was there, one of the larger boys had just brought in a bucket of fresh water from the well. I was supposed to put several drops of Clorox into each bucket of well water before anyone went to the back of the room to get their tin cup to get a drink. While I was talking with Nurse Johnson, the local health inspector showed up and tested the water. No Clorox in the water! I received my first reprimand, a severe rebuke. Needless to say, I was crushed. Miss Johnson came to my rescue and told the inspector that I was busy talking to her and had not had time to put Clorox in the water. I don't think he apologized, but he sure should have. And I never again failed to keep an eagle eye on the water pail. The water pail provided a few other adventures. Some of the children would invariably forget to use their tin cup and would drink from the dipper. I strongly encouraged them to never do it again.

Hilda Snider, "Hilda Snider Recalls Teaching at Mitchell Run,"
Reflections, *February 2006*

Contaminated Water

The open well at Peddler Gap School was contaminated with a dog that was put in the well by someone that thought it was a suitable Halloween prank. Water had to be carried from a neighbor's house, but it was working alive with wiggle tails (mosquito larvae).

The neighbor's husband caught two catfish and put them in the well and sure enough those catfish ate the mosquitoes.

Jimmie Jones, West Liberty, December 29, 2008

Vernacular Bible

We always started school every morning by singing "America," then made a pledge to the flag, and then a scripture verse.

One little boy got up one morning and said, "If you mind your mammy and your pappy, you won't get a whipping." [*Laughter*]

He was referring to a Bible verse.

Duval Sidebottom Hay, Campbellsville, December 11, 2008

Teacher's Sisters

I have one little funny thing I'd like to share. During my first year of teaching I had my two younger sisters in school. Everybody packed their lunch, and maybe once a week my mother was able to buy a loaf of white bread. Otherwise, my sisters took biscuits to school with them. The biscuits had ham, jelly, or a fried egg between them.

On the days that my sisters had their sandwiches made from loaf bread, they would eat in the schoolhouse. On the days they had biscuits, they would always go outside to eat, no matter how cold it was. They seemed to be embarrassed by bringing homemade bread to school.

My, my, it took an industrious woman to get up and make enough biscuits for a family of seven, with enough left over to make sandwiches for school.

On the last day of school we had a field day, competing in running relays, jumping, etc. My youngest sister was an excellent athlete, placing first in all the contests, but I would never give the prize to her. Instead I always awarded it to the second-place winner.

I felt it would not look good on either one of us. The other sister would always promise her something to not cry or make a scene. To this day she reminds me from time to time of all that bubblegum and stick candy she won fair and square!

Betty Jo Arnett Lykins, Salyersville, February 1, 2009

Field Trip for the War Effort

This happened back during World War II, and scrap iron was a great big thing. So they asked the schools to bring scrap iron. So my dad hitched two mules to the wagon one morning, and I drove that to school, loaded up the children, then went around and got a big load of scrap iron.

I went and unloaded that, then went again. So I got two loads of scrap iron that day. Some of the children would walk along; some of them would ride on the back pole. There wasn't any danger of anybody getting hurt. We just had fun collecting scrap iron, and enjoyed eating lunch, which we took with us. It was a picnic all day.

Duval Sidebottom Hay, Campbellsville, December 11, 2008

Teacher's Pet

At Sharon School there were two doors on the front of the building, one of which was for girls and the other one for boys. Girls sat on one side of the school and boys on the other. There were also separate outhouses for boys and girls

There was one little girl there who was the "teacher's pet." She was really too young to attend school, but stayed there the whole year. She was cute and had to be excused to go outside and "dawdle" frequently.

I'll never forget her being there that year.

Martha Campbell, Central City, December 13, 2008

How Times Have Changed

This is something that took place while I was teaching at Fairview. The thing that happened did not seem unusual until modern times. A brother of some of the students was out hunting rabbits and stopped by the school. He asked for permission to visit his sister and brothers for a few minutes.

He had a gun with him, so I asked him to unload his gun and leave his dead rabbits and gun out on the porch. He did what I asked, then came in, visited quietly, and left.

Basically that was a nonevent, as no one gave it a second thought. However, today the mere mention of a gun near school is cause for panic. My, how times have changed.

William H. Nicholls Jr., The Villages, Fla., December 14, 2008

Gun Play

Back when I was teaching I considered myself a crack shot with a rifle. I took my .22 rifle with me to school and at recess I taught the boys how to shoot. Most likely, doing that at school wouldn't fly these days.

However, I find it interesting that in current times there is a shooting sports class at Lyon County High School, and girls are also included.

Hale Murphy, Eddyville, December 31, 2008

Never Mind

This little girl lived with her grandparents, and she got upset about something there at school. She said to me, "Miss Anna, I'm going home."

I said, "If you want to go home, you go right ahead, but you know what will happen as soon as you get home?"

She said, "Yes."

I said, "What will happen?"

She said, "They'll send me right back."

I said, "Well, it doesn't make much sense to go home, does it?"

Then she said, "No, I think I'll just stay here." [*Laughter*]

Something had upset her, but I don't remember what it was. Let me say, teaching is a wonderful profession, but you'd better like it.

Anna Smith Collins, Marion, November 20, 2008

Better Things to Do

I don't remember what grade he was in, but this boy got up and started to leave school. I had to go get him. I asked him why he was leaving, and he said he had better things to do at home.

Well, I brought him back, but he didn't try to put up an excuse for leaving.

Velois S. Fitts, Winchester, as told to Deborah Evans Colburn,
March 17, 2009

Becoming Christian

A few years ago one of my former female students called and said that she wanted to thank me for her Christianity.

She was talking about the fact that during a revival at church, the student body went as a group to a morning revival service on a school day, and she became a Christian that day.

Hale Murphy, Eddyville, December 31, 2008

Helpful Advice

At one particular school [as a substitute teacher], I struggled through a week of fixing soup on the stove and then having to use that same soup pot in which to heat water, wash bowls and spoons. I mentioned to one of the watching children that I didn't know how the regular teacher managed to do all that.

The little girl looked at me with puzzlement and replied, "Oh, she don't never wash the dishes here. She takes them home with her at night."

Norma Ramsey Eversole, Mt. Vernon, January 9, 2009

Overloaded Teacher

My fourth year of teaching was at a school in Windy, also here in Wayne County. In years past the school building had been a high school, but now most of the high school building was torn down. Only the part needed for the grade school was left. It was in pretty good condition though, and the rooms were spacious. There were forty-eight students and I was the only teacher. I really had to use the older students to help with the younger students.

There wasn't much time for each class, so I had to go in a run all day long. I developed a nervous disorder for which I was taking medicine by the end of the year.

Lucille Hoover Ringley, Monticello, March 24, 2007

Student Reset the Clock

At Breezeel School I had lots of trouble working in all the subjects for all grades. At first I started the day where I left off the day before. Each class came to the benches at the front of the room for the lessons.

I used a small alarm clock that I could see from my desk. One day I found myself way behind with the classes. What happened, this big boy had run the clock up an hour as he sat on the bench for class. I dismissed early and moved the clock.

Mattie Jo Smith, Benton, March 7, 2009

Frog Comes to Class

I had a second-grade boy who went to the branch below school and caught a frog. He brought it into the schoolroom and put it in his desk.

We were having classes and the frog hopped out onto the floor and was hopping around the classroom. This was amusing to everyone.

Kolema Stearns Davis, Taylorsville, February 6, 2009

THE SCARY MAN AND THE CRAZY MAN

One of my first graders, Ann, was very timid and didn't expect anyone to visit our little Douglas School. We had no telephone, so teachers weren't notified by the Pike County School central office when a supervisor or an attendance officer was coming to visit. One very busy day in walked Mr. Prater, the attendance officer. He began talking to the students about the importance of attending school. While he was talking I heard giggles. I looked over at the little wooden table where my five first graders sat and immediately noticed Betty really giggling. I waited until Mr. Prater left, then I asked, "Betty, why are you giggling?"

She answered, "Look under the table and see Ann."

I looked, and there saw Ann hunkered underneath. I asked her, "Why are you under the table?"

With tears in her eyes, she responded, "Miss Thacker, that big man looked scary."

I encouraged her by saying, "Please come out and sit in your chair. We don't need to be scared. Mr. Prater is one of our friends, and he travels to various schools to see how we are doing. He will come several times to visit us because he loves children."

Within two weeks from that day, the whole class had a very scary experience—not only the children, but for me too. One of the older students looked out the window and saw an elderly man coming out of the forest at the edge of our school ground. The student said, "Miss Thacker, look! I see a real old man that is walking like a drunken man. Come here and look."

The other students and I hurried to the window. Two of the students, Lisa and Melody, quickly recognized him because their father was his landlord. They said, "Oh, that is Mr. Jacob, and he is crazy. Daddy told us how he has been acting and that his two sons, Bryan and Kevin, had to watch their daddy all the time." Apparently Mr. Jacob had been slipping off, causing his sons to keep a close eye on him. He had already walked about one-half mile to get to our school ground. The students said, "Miss Thacker, close the door. He is crazy and dangerous." I, too, had heard this rumor, but didn't dare say, "He is crazy."

I quickly closed the door. We were afraid to look out the front door because Mr. Jacob might be there on the steps. Concerned for my students' safety, I explained, "If anyone needs to go to the toilet, I'll help you out the window." (During those days no one- or two-room schools had indoor plumbing.) We tried to continue our assignments and activities like normal, but did not know if or when it would be safe for us to leave the building. I felt frightened! I had a great responsibility to care for my students and keep them in a calm atmosphere.

Ten or fifteen minutes later some of the students were looking out the window and saw the man's two sons following the same path Mr. Jacob had walked. They went around to the back of the building. Feeling much better, I said, "Oh, there are Mr. Jacob's sons. Let's hope they can rescue their dear old daddy before he gets on the highway." A few minutes later we saw the two sons trying to lead their disturbed father back around the school towards his home. Mr. Jacob was really resisting them and was trying to get loose. We quickly felt a sigh of relief as we watched his sons take him back down the path at the edge of the school ground.

Later on we learned Mr. Jacob had become so mentally disturbed within a few days after our frightful day that his family admitted him to the Eastern Kentucky Mental Hospital in Lexington. Unfortunately he lived only a few days there before passing away.

I don't know if any of my students, other than Lisa and Melody who recognized Mr. Jacob, had ever heard people say, "He or she has gone crazy." I think the word "crazy" was used mostly in the eastern portion of the state. The folks in my home community always spoke of the person as crazy, and never used the word insane. People also would say their family will have to send that person to Lexington to the asylum.

To this day I still have vivid memories of this elderly insane man who walked one-half mile to my school ground, and how frightened we were.

Christine Thacker Justice, Mt. Sterling, February 18, 2009

First Paycheck Well Spent

All of the one- or two-room schools in Kentucky had no indoor plumbing and each one used a potbelly stove for heat. No janitorial service was provided. Each teacher was responsible for keeping their classroom clean and for building fires in the stove. Therefore, most of the teachers hired, from their own personal funds, one of their older or dependable students to do these tasks. Of course teachers only hired someone to be the janitor during the cold weather months, as cleaning during the other months didn't require too much effort. You had to be very careful as to the student you hired as the janitor, because you issued them the school building's key.

From 1940 to 1942 my twin sister and I were students at Sims Creek. Mrs. Cool, our seventh- and eighth-grade teacher, hired my sister, Ernestine, and me to be her janitors. We gladly accepted the tasks, as earning ten cents a day sounded great! Our parents had taught us to be thrifty.

After my sister and I began working we soon decided what we would purchase with our very first two-dollar paycheck. We had been dreaming about getting a much-needed dictionary each, as we only got to use the one dictionary that Mrs. Cool kept on her desk. We knew that we could increase our vocabulary if we had our own personal dictionary. When Mrs. Cool handed us the two dollars at the end of the month (twenty school days at ten cents), we felt happy. We knew that was enough to buy two dictionaries. We said to the teacher, "Mrs. Cool, would you please take this money and purchase each of us a dictionary?"

She answered, "I don't drive to Pikeville very often. It will probably be about a month." We anxiously waited a few weeks for our dictionaries. One Monday morning Mrs. Cool walked up to her desk and said, "Ernestine and Christine, please come here." We gladly walked up to the desk, where she presented us the two new dictionaries. I used that dictionary throughout my high school and college years.

I will always remember and appreciate how that janitor job helped us financially.

Christine Thacker Justice, Mt. Sterling, February 18, 2009

Chapter 5

Disciplining Students

Although Kentucky's one-room school teachers emphasize that showing respect for one's elders was in their day a common expectation held of children, they also recognize that it is in the nature of children to misbehave occasionally. Times were different then, and disciplinary methods considered unacceptable today were the norm. The paddle, the switch, the ruler, or the teacher's bare hand were commonly employed to make an impression on misbehaving students—and generally the students preferred that method to lecturing. Usually, but not always, parents supported teachers in these situations.

Corporal Punishment

When I was teaching at Gregory School, I had been threatening to discipline this little boy. One day he did something bad enough that I thought he needed spanking. So I just pulled him down across my lap and took my hand and spanked him really hard. It was hard enough that he felt it.

He had on a new pair of overalls, and they caused me to almost blister my hand! When I felt that, I stopped! [*Laughter*]

Students back then knew when they needed spanking. They might not admit it, but they knew what to expect.

Alma New, Monticello, November 7, 2008

Miss Priss the Wildcat

I used to get spankings in first grade all the time. I talked when I would get on the floor. I was just Little Miss Priss. I'd get up and prance around! The teacher would spank me, but I didn't get mad because I knew I deserved to be spanked.

I was a wildcat!!

Georgia Lloyd, Barbourville, November 21, 2008

Whipping with an Extra Lick

My sister and I had a fight at school once. Something happened between my sister and this boy that we called Dove. I think he shoved her down and they started fighting. His sister started taking up for him, and when she jumped in I started taking up for my sister. We fought and fought, and when we went inside we had to take our medicine.

I had never been whipped at school in my life and didn't think I ever would be. Anyway, the teacher gave each one two licks. I was last, and when she gave me two licks I was pretty sassy. I turned around and said, "That's enough; that's all you gave her."

Then she gave me another lick! I really did get whipped!

Laura Agnes Townsley Stacy, Barbourville, November 21, 2008

Alpha Dog

One day [Keith] got up and defied me in front of the whole group [of students]. I thought, "This is it. I've got to be the winner. I've got to be the alpha dog here; no doubt about it!" I'd give him every opportunity, and they all saw what I was doing. I didn't take him back in the room by himself to spank him. But I did spank him with a paddle, wore him out. He went around and around, and I did too. My arm was worn out by the time I spanked him three times, but I don't think I bruised him at all because the next morning he was sitting on the steps. I couldn't believe it, but I walked up to that school, and there he sat. I thought, "My God, he's going to whip me. What will I do?" I thought that because he was bigger than I was.

When I walked up he said, "Good morning Mrs. Goodin."

I said, "Good morning, Keith. How are you?"

He said, "I'm okay. I'm sorry about yesterday. Would you care if I built your fires from now on?"

I said, "Oh, Keith, that would be wonderful," and then I went to him and hugged him around the neck. He was my slave from then on. I felt he needed attention, and I guess I gave him all he needed.

Daphne H. Goodin, Barbourville, November 21, 2008

Unexpected Paddling

The kids I can remember giving a good paddling to in a one-room school were at Big Creek. These two boys were either seventh or eighth graders, and they were two of my good basketball players, but they were always aggravating the girls and the little boys. They'd always say, "Alright, I'm going to get you in a minute," and just kept on.

One day it just hit me, so I grabbed my paddle and made them both bend over, and I mean I fired their bottoms! Well, a Ferquin boy got just as pale as a sheep. He was fair colored, but he got so pale. He turned around and said, "I can't believe you did that."

I said, "I told you I was going to."

Then they said, "Yes, but we didn't believe you." [*Laughter*]

Virginia Janes, Edmonton, September 22, 2008

Teacher Rules

I didn't spank my students, because they never needed to be spanked. In those days, instead of spanking you ruled their hands. I would take hold of their hand and hold it tight, then take a ruler and just hit it. That was my way of making them mind and not misbehave.

If they really needed to be disciplined, I would stand them in the corner, with their face in the corner, or I would make them write a poem of something, so many times.

I don't remember what all I did to punish them, but with nothing severe. The children in those days were so different. I mean, they just showed me they loved me to death. They always called me "Miss Mayola."

I have students to this day that I taught in the 1930s and early 1940s to come see me, send me cards, and call me. That is precious to me.

Mayola Graves, Loretto, September 9, 2008

Apology for Bad Behavior

Very seldom did I ever have to punish students, but here is a story about the time I did have to do it. The students were out of the schoolhouse after lunch one afternoon, and I saw an eighth grade boy aggravating a little second- or third-grade boy. So I went over and said to the eighth-grade boy, "James, march yourself into the classroom right now."

So he went in and, of course, I went in too. I went to my desk, and he went to his desk. At that time we had bottles of ink and an ink staff with a point in it.

I looked up and he was holding that bottle of ink up like he was going to throw it at me. I said, "Just go on and throw it, James." Instead of telling him not to, I said, "Throw it."

When I said that, he just sat down. He didn't throw it!

When he got ready to go home that afternoon, I wrote a note to his parents that said, "One of you must accompany James to school in the morning, and he must apologize to me for his behavior."

One parent came with him. When James apologized, he just told me that he was sorry that he first bothered the little boy, then he went on to say, "I'm sorry I picked up that bottle of ink and I'm glad I didn't throw it."

Back then we had very, very few discipline problems with students. It is so different now, as parents will often sue the teacher or principal.

Mayola Graves, Loretto, September 9, 2008

Two Bad Brothers

There were a couple of boys at Oak Hill that were kind of rough customers. Their names were Edward and Mitchell Ferguson, and they caused me a little bit of trouble. I had to talk pretty rough to them sometimes. I'd stand them in the corner of the room and talk to them to get them to behave. But I never did spank them.

J. Robert Miller, Rock Bridge, September 18, 2008

Helpful Delinquent

I had an unruly boy during my first teaching year. He disobeyed a rule, and just wouldn't do what he was told to do.

I said, "Well, you know what you do, and what you'll get if you can't follow the rule. You'll either go home, or you'll get a whipping."

Believe it or not, he went outside and got a switch and brought it in and handed it to me.

I hit him about twice! [*Laughter*]

Blanche Demunbrun, Glasgow, September 30, 2008

Few Troubles

Students back then were always respectful of teachers, and it was the same way when I went to a one-room school at Merryville in Monroe County.

I don't remember ever spanking a student. But if they did something that should not have happened, I made them sit in a corner there in the room to be isolated. They didn't like that, so that was punishment enough.

They had to sit there in the corner for ten or fifteen minutes, maybe until their class was called to order and it was time for them to recite. At that point they could come out of the corner.

Back then children weren't misbehaving like kids in school now do. They'd get into little squabbles on the playground, picking on each other, writing on each other's paper to just mess it up, but they pretty well settled the problems themselves. I would separate them just to make sure they did.

On occasion, if they got into a fight, I'd move them from the back of the schoolroom up to the front seat, and they didn't like that.

I don't remember ever having a student that was a constant troublemaker.

Betty Jane (Miller) Pence, Franklin, Tenn., September 29, 2008

Unusual, but Effective, Form of Discipline

One thing that I had dealt with was one family that lived down on the river. I never did know them until I had to go stay all night with them. Their girls had rocked the schoolhouse by throwing rocks on it, so I went to their house to calm them down.

After I spent that night with them, that was it. They didn't do it again.

Their girls rocked the schoolhouse because I had stayed all night with some of the other children, and they did this to make me stay all night with them.

At least they did it to have me stay with them.

Blanche Demunbrun, Glasgow, September 30, 2008

Not How We Use a Compass

Some teachers spanked kids every now and then, but I never was one that believed in that. I always said, "If I have to spank a lot, I'll find myself a different profession."

But there were a few times during my first four years in Sano at Bryant School when I had this little seventh grader that decided to use his compass and stick the bottom end of it in the student in front of him!

Well, I did give him a little punishment.

Zona Royse, Columbia, October 4, 2008

Lesson Learned

I never shall forget this. I had said something to one of the parents about the school building and that it sure did need to be painted. That was the last year I was there. I don't know whether they had in mind to consolidate that school as soon as they did or not. Anyway, the school board agreed to have the building painted.

Well, I was so thrilled to go back to school and see the building painted white. It looked so nice and clean. Well, it rained one afternoon, and I let the students out for recess. Two of my little girls had an old rubber sponge ball, and they thought they would throw this ball at the side of the building. Of course, part of the time they didn't catch the sponge ball, and it got mud on it.

I went out, and the side of the building was polky-dot, with streams of mud going down this freshly painted building. I thought, "How can I face the people in this community? What on earth will they think of me?"

Well, I took the two little girls inside the building and I talked to them. After that, I talked to the whole room of students. I said, "Now, I'm going to spank both of you. You both knew better than to do that. How are you going to feel when people come by and say, 'Look at all that mud on the side of that building, and it was just recently painted.'"

I really got onto them; tore up their conscience, so I guess I did preach a good sermon. Anyway, I spanked both of them in front of the whole room of students. I said, "Now, let this be a lesson to all of you. This is not my nature to have to spank children, but when my own disobeyed me, they suffered the consequences. So this is one time right here that you're going to have to learn to make choices in life, and try to make the right decisions on what is right, and what is wrong."

Well, I had perfect discipline after that. Nobody dared to do anything wrong after that.

Back to the two girls, I made them get a bucket of water, and we did have a ladder in the cloakroom. Well, as far as they could reach up on that building, I made those two girls scrub those ball spots down.

Some of the older boys could reach up higher, and I think I even brought a ladder from home, a long ladder. I got my son Bill, who was in the eighth grade, up there on it and he cleaned the rest of it down.

So I saved my face in the public eye by removing the polky-dot mud from the building. After that we had a good school year.

One of these two girls was in a family of twelve children, and I had five of them at the same time in different grades. One of the little girls that threw the ball was Bonnie, and I saw her not too long ago. Of course, she's a mother and grandmother now. She looked at me and said, "Miss Emma, I'll never forget that whipping."

I said, "And you know why?"

She said, "Wasn't that the dumbest thing for me to do something like that?"

I said, "Well, that's the reason I gave you both a spanking. I wanted to make an impression on you that you must learn to make right choices, and when you make wrong choices, you're going to suffer consequences."

She said, "Oh, I found that out so many times in life."

Emma Walker, Eddyville, October 7, 2008

Cleaning Columbus

I hung up a picture of Christopher Columbus on the wall at school. Some of the boys had taken some mud balls and threw them at the picture. I asked them why they had done that, and they told me they didn't like the picture. I told them to figure out how to reach the picture and get up there to clean up their mess. They scurried off to a nearby home to get a ladder. Then they cleaned up their mess, and they never caused me another problem.

They deserved it, but I never did spank any of the children at school.

Loella Lowery, as told to Jeannine Moore, Dawson Springs,
January 10, 2009

Geography Lesson

I forget the boy's name, but he had been coming to school. His daddy would come up on Friday afternoons to play ball, and finally he took a group of boys down to Sand Lick. He didn't ask for my permission to take them in his truck, and I didn't hardly know how to punish all of them. However, I do remember that I used the big green geography book to do the spanking.

Mamie Wright, Tompkinsville, October 16, 2008

Cheater

I remember that I had one girl who was so bad to cheat. I'd catch her cheating all the time, and I'd take her paper away from her. I'd give it back to her later and tell her to straighten it out and do it herself. She had brothers and sisters there, too, and a lot of times they'd tell on her.

As to how she cheated, let's say that if she were doing math, she'd cheat off somebody else, then hold her hand up to give the answer! [*Laughter*]

If I'd see her cheating, or if the kids would tell on her by saying, "Dessie is cheating," I'd take her paper away from her.

But I never did spank children for anything like that. I don't know why, but I just never did.

Virginia Janes, Edmonton, September 22, 2008

Spankings

I hardly ever spanked girls. I remember a girl that needed it, but I was afraid that this girl would go home and tell her parents that she'd been spanked. I always wanted to do something that would impress her parents, but in this case I was afraid her parents would accuse me of not being the right kind of teacher.

Colonel Benton Bowman was one of the students that I spanked, and I'll never forget he had the fattest little bottom I can remember. The parents of boys didn't mind me spanking their boys, because they'd tell them if they got a spanking at school, they would spank them also when they got home.

Mamie Wright, Tompkinsville, October 16, 2008

FAST-RUNNING MISCREANT

This is a discipline problem story that took place during the second year I taught at a one-room school called Missouri Hollow. That year I had forty-six or forty-seven children in that school; thus there wasn't hardly enough room for all of them in that building.

One family had four children there, three sons and a daughter. Since they lived just down the road a little ways from the school, their children went home for lunch each day.

Well, that morning just as I drove into the playground at school, two boys were already there, and they were fighting. They both had rocks in their hands ready to throw at each other. I jumped out of the car quickly and said, "Drop those rocks *right now!*"

One of them did very nicely put the rocks down, but the other one hauled off and threw a rock and hit the other boy as hard as he could. Well, I took off chasing him, as I was going to wear him out, and I did. After I chased him down and caught him, I just wore him out with a paddle.

He went home for lunch, and his mother came back to school with him. She was very upset that I had spanked him. However, she never would come up into the playground. She stayed right there in the road, then asked me to come down so she could talk to me. So I stepped down away from the playground and went down toward her. Then she told me that she didn't appreciate me spanking her son because he hadn't done so-and-so, so-and-so, and so-and-so.

I explained to her what her son had done and why I had spanked him. Then she said, "Well, I'll just tell you, I thought about not sending my children up here, because they tell me there is nothing but hoodlums that comes to school up here!"

I said, "Mrs. Brummett, that's not nice of you to call the children hoodlums. Now remember, you have four that's coming here, and when you refer to all of them like that, you are referring to your own children, and that is not nice."

So we went on and discussed matters for quite a while. She never did come up on the playground, and I never did go down to the road where she was standing. We continued discussing things, but before we finished she apologized to me, saying, "I'm sorry that I've come up here to do this, but I'll tell you why I am so mad." (Her little boy's name was David.) "Every time I try to spank him, he runs off from me, and I cannot catch him. You have caught him and spanked him, and that's made me mad because I can't catch him." [*Laughter*]

Her husband had a wooden leg, and he couldn't do any discipline or anything, so she had to do all of it, and that was why she was so angry with me.

I'll have to say that David was one of the best children I had for the rest of that year. I never had another bit of trouble, but children did have to obey what I asked them to do.

Wanda Humble, Monticello, November 7, 2008

Head Start

This is a discipline story. Sometimes parents in the community were a little agitated with each other. When I was teaching at Cedar Hill, I had two families that could not get along. They were always bickering back and forth, so that carried over to the school. Their kids had to walk home from school on the same road, and it finally got so bad that I decided, after consulting with their parents, that I'd dismiss the family that always gets the bad end of it on their trip home every day, fifteen minutes early every day.

That would get these kids a good ways along up the hill before this other bunch of children got out. So, that was well and good, and I told this mother when she came down, "This is what we're going to do, so if your children dillydally around and don't get on home, and this other group catches up with them, that's going to be their fault."

As far as I know, that worked. I never heard any more about that problem.

Imogene Dick, Monticello, November 7, 2008

PECULIAR DISCIPLINARY ACTION

I didn't really do a lot of spanking. It was just more like making the student stand in the corner of the room with their face pointed toward the corner, or taking recess away from them, and doing things like that. I can even remember making students stand with their nose in a ring [circle] on the blackboard.

I don't remember what the problem was, but that was one of the ways I disciplined them if they didn't do what they were supposed to do. I just took them up to the board, drew a ring on the board, and they had to stand there with their nose in the ring until I told them to sit down. The length of time they had to stand there with their nose in the ring depended on how roughly they had acted, I guess. It was typically not more than five or ten minutes.

I'm sure that one of my teachers did that, or I would have never thought of it.

Wanda Humble, Monticello, November 7, 2008

RING PUNISHMENT

I usually didn't spank kids. Sometimes I would if I had told them several times to not do something. But I usually just made them stand in the corner of the room, which would embarrass them more than anything.

Or I would draw a circle on the board, then make them stand up there with their nose inside the circle, or ring, as we called it.

Joyce Williams Ward, Campbellsville, December 11, 2008

NOT READY FOR SCHOOL

I remember spanking a little boy that was in first grade and a large boy for not doing their work. The first grader would come to school, but would go home for lunch with all his other brothers and sisters. After they had eaten lunch, he would come back and play in the mountain the rest of the afternoon.

He wouldn't come on back to school, and when I sent the report cards home that year, his mother couldn't understand his failure. His brothers and sisters told their mother that he was just not in attendance, that he had been going to the mountain in the afternoon to play in a big sagebrush field. He wasn't ready for school.

His parents didn't come to talk with me about their son. They just listened to the word of the other children. The next year he did fine.

Joyce Campbell Buchanan, Barbourville, November 21, 2008

BALER TWINE DISCIPLINE

I got baler twine from our farm and took it to school. My chief way to discipline was using baler twine. A little first grader that couldn't sit in his seat didn't know how to sit in it because they didn't have chairs at home. They didn't have a place to sit; they squatted.

A lot of the other kids didn't have a place to sit, so they just stood at the tables at home. One reason they wanted to come to school was because it was warm and clean and they could sit down.

I would take my baler twine and say, "Now, this is your seat and your desk that you're responsible for." And I would tie them to the seat with the twine and say, "If you need to get up, just pull this string and let it drop apart, but don't pull that string unless it is necessary." Then, I'd show them and have them practice so they would know what to do. And if I had two kids that got into a fight, I'd tie their two left hands together with a string. That way, you are your brother's keeper, or your sister's keeper, even your cousin's keeper.

I don't think I ever tied two people together more than once a day. Usually, about two months in school most of the baler twine just hung up on the wall. During the first month I had taught them what I expected them to do.

Those kids truly loved me. . . .

One little boy gave me a lot of problems, so I tied him to the stove by himself. I made him lie down under the stove, and then tied one of his arms to the one leg of the stove, and another to the other stove leg. Then I said to him, "Now, you can take your teeth and open the string and get out from under there." He was under the stove on the floor because he was uncontrollable.

The next day when I rode my horse into the schoolyard, there stood his father. I was still on my horse when he said, "I hear that you tied my son and made him lie on the floor."

Even though they squatted on the floor, they would never sit on the floor. That was taboo, as the floor was dirty.

I made him lie on the floor and I tied him. The father asked me about that, and I said, "Yes, I did that."

He looked at me and said, "Well, you are first one that has ever made him obey. Keep it up." Then he walked away! [*Laughter*]

Irma Gall, Barbourville, November 20, 2008

Respect Your Elders

In high school I had a history teacher who was also my neighbor, and I was being a smart aleck. I talked back to her, then she said, "Alright, young lady, I'll talk with your parents."

She went out and over to Daddy's store and talked to my mother and daddy, and I got a spanking over that! My parents wore me out. They said, "You don't ever talk back to a teacher; you show respect."

Daddy was awful bad about that, and he would say, "You are supposed to respect an elder, no matter what."

After class that day I said to the teacher, "You know what you caused me to get—a spanking, and I'll never like you again."

She grabbed me and hugged me and said, "Georgia, you love me," and I said, "Yeah, I do."

Georgia Lloyd, Barbourville, November 21, 2008

Fight between Boy and Teacher

One day I knew that something was up relative to this one eighth-grade boy. I ate my lunch at my desk and went outside. Just as I got outside, he jumped on me from the corner. He was going to whip me like he did the others. I grabbed him and threw him right down through a briar patch. It really skinned him. I'd be in jail today for the rest of my life for doing that. But that's all it took that one time.

Pat McDonald, Barbourville, November 21, 2008

First Spanking

After I first started teaching, I guess it was three or four weeks before I spanked anybody. Finally, three or four girls got into a little fight. The parents had already been down checking on me and wondered why I hadn't spanked anybody, and things like that.

I had a little twelve-inch ruler on my desk, but never did have a paddle. Anyway, these little girls were in about third or fourth grade, and I made a decision to spank them in their hands. I bent their hands back and gave them two or three little swats. That was the first spanking I ever remember giving a child in school.

There's a lady here in Knox County that reminds me of that spanking. She tells me that I gave her a spanking! [*Laughter*]

I never did really believe in paddling kids that much. I spanked kids a little bit more after that, but not a lot. I did spank some of the boys on their bottoms. To do that, I had them to lean over so I could spank them on the rear, but I never did spank girls on the butt. I always spanked them in the hand.

I usually used my hands when spanking the boys, but sometimes used a little paddle.

The kids didn't get mad at me when I spanked them, but on one occasion a little boy did get angry. Typically I didn't make it too hard on them.

Sometimes after I did a spanking, some other kids would laugh. When they did this I also spanked them! They weren't allowed to do that.

Bige R. Warren, Barbourville, November 20, 2008

Stuck to the Seat

My first spanking was for two fourth-grade boys who were fighting. I paddled the first boy, but the second boy held onto his seat and wouldn't move.

I talked to his parents and they came to school the next day to witness the whipping, but the boy still would not move from his seat. I gave him a few licks on his legs while he was still in his seat.

I never had any more trouble with this boy. Any time girls or boys got into a fight, I paddled both of them.

Michael M. Meredith, Bee Spring, December 7, 2008

Teacher Wanted; Climbing Skills Required

Old Salem School was in the neighborhood where my grandmother lived across the Green River from where I lived. I thought I wouldn't take that job when it was offered to me because I wanted to go back to school, but Superintendent Mrs. Burris said, "I'm desperate."

I found out that the first teacher they had wasn't liked by any of the children, so they turned her horse loose and let it go home. Then they got the second teacher, but the children didn't like her either, so they locked her up in the well house. Then I was their third teacher. Well, I went in and took a bunch of magazines and played with the children and got on their good side! I had no trouble from them.

I had five first cousins [as students] while teaching at Old Salem. One day my cousin Bobby got mad at me and he went out and climbed a tree. He said, "If you want me, you'll come and get me."

Well, that didn't bother me a bit because I could skin up a tree like anybody else! So I went up the tree and he kept kicking back and forth. I tried to get hold of his britches and finally did, so I just pulled him down. Tree limbs were breaking, and he was hollering, "Don't do that! Don't do that!"

When we got down out of the tree I took him inside and then said to him, "Now, Bobby, I'm not going to put up with that. We're going to act like we're supposed to, and you're going to be a better boy."

He said, "I'm going to tell my mama when I get home."

I said, "No, you're not. I'm going to tell her when we get there."

On the way home that day he said, "Miss Duval, if you won't tell my mother, I'll forget about it, and we won't ever talk about it anymore."

I said, "No, I'm going to tell her," and I did. His mother got a board and spanked his bottom and put him in a chair.

The next day at school I had no trouble at all. Everybody was afraid the teacher was going to get the best of them, I guess.

Duval Sidebottom Hay, Campbellsville, December 11, 2008

Behavior Turnaround

When I started teaching at Farmers there was a great big boy in the seventh grade. I guess he was six feet tall. They told me, "You'll probably have trouble with him because he runs off every teacher that comes here to teach, or he gives them trouble."

People at the office told me, "If he gives you trouble, tell us and we'll expel him."

I think there were five children in that family in school there. He hadn't really done anything to me, but everyday he'd manage to slip around and eat all of his little sisters' lunch. And here we'd go to lunch, but they didn't have any lunch. I knew what was happening, but I never could catch him. He was just big, and very hungry.

I was agitated over that with him, but couldn't catch him. One Friday afternoon was the first time he ever did a smart aleck thing to me. I had five seventh graders, and I was doing something with them, and I handed him his paper and pencil and something. He jerked it away and acted real smart alecky. Well, we had a table there that had some little logs on it, as we were building a cabinet. I picked one of the logs up and just whammed him over the shoulder as hard as I could. Then I said to him, "I want to tell you something. If you want to come up here to school and behave, I want to see you back; otherwise, I don't want you on this school ground."

Tears came into his eyes, and I thought to myself, "Boy, I've had it! He'll cut the tires off of my car, or he'll do something to me."

When I got to school on Monday he was sweeping the floor. When I got there the next day he gave me an apple! I didn't have any more trouble with him. He was smart, and if he wanted to do something about his study, he could do it. He had plenty of intelligence.

Years later, after the schools were consolidated, the director of pupil personnel came to me. She was out from that area, and she knew the story. She said to me, "I have had a request from some company in Indiana wanting a recommendation about this particular student, and I figure you probably got more out of him than anybody else, and he probably stayed at school longer to you than anybody else. What can you say good about him?"

I said, "Tell them that if he wants to do it, he can do it."

Duval Sidebottom Hay, Campbellsville, December 11, 2008

Peach Offering

At Lone Oak School there was a little room in which we kept our coats and water buckets and other things. The door was always open to the school, so before I got there one morning there was a group of schoolchildren there roughhousing in the little room. They had literally destroyed some school property.

When I went in I asked who destroyed things, but no one confessed. I said, "Well, we'll just get you all." So I spanked every one of them. I don't remember how many there were, but I spanked them all.

One of the children that went home for lunch told his mother that

I had spanked him that morning. So they spent the afternoon trying to get him into another school. There were two other schools available for him to go to, but for some reason they couldn't get him admitted to either of those schools. So he decided to come on back to me.

The next morning when he came to school, he had a peach that must have been six inches in diameter. I had never seen such a large peach. That was his peace offering, and he never gave me another minute of trouble at all, and his family didn't.

He later went away, got married, then came back several years ago. When I would see him out, he always told me I was one of his favorite teachers and would go on to say something good about me.

He died about three years ago with cancer, but he was on my good side. I can't forget that peach. It was the biggest peach I ever saw.

Bernadine Shirley Sullivan, Campbellsville, December 11, 2008

Correcting Misbehaving Students

If an argument or fight happened on the playground, I took those involved into the cloakroom so that each one could tell their side of the story. Usually the fight was between friends or close "buddies," and they would have to say to each other that they were sorry, then shake hands and spend the rest of the playtime sitting in their seats inside the classroom.

When an incident happened inside during classes, I took the guilty one or ones out in the hall and we discussed their behavior. I asked them if they weren't embarrassed and they usually replied, "Yes."

On one occasion I told a first grader he must cooperate with me, or I would spank him. He fell into my arms and replied, "Mrs. Bailey, if you'll tell me what that means, I'll do it." I didn't spank, but explained the meaning to him.

Garnet Gay Bailey Goble, Flat Gap, January 20, 2009

Guilty Conscience

Discipline in both one-room schools in which I taught was at a minimum. The only spanking I ever did was to Brownie Goodin, who had a hot temper. I don't remember why I spanked him, but it took care of the problem.

That same day on my way home from school, and thinking about how I hated to spank Brownie, a green snake crossed my path. Being deathly afraid of snakes, I thought seeing that snake was punishment for my spanking Brownie.

Grace W. McGaughey, Lexington, January 29, 2009

CRUEL AND UNUSUAL PUNISHMENT

On Halloween night the boys used to get out and do some mischievous things like turning the girls' outdoor toilet upside down. Well, one of the girls went to the outside toilet the morning after Halloween, and the toilet was turned upside down. She went running back to the house and said, "There's a snake in the toilet." Well, that was something!

Then the boys grabbed their slugger bats and started running to the toilet. That was the end of those chicken snakes, and they have never been seen since. It really was a snake located up on the rafter. I guess the boys had put the snake up there!

I think it was Lynwood, Charles, and Wallace that turned the toilet upside down! [*Laughter*] I didn't punish them for doing that, but I think I let them sit in my lap for the rest of the day. Sitting in my lap was enough punishment for what they did!

Mamie Wright, Tompkinsville, October 16, 2008

MAMA AND TEACHER BOTH SPANK

Mama was a good teacher, actually my best teacher. This is about an incident that took place when I was in the fourth or fifth grade. This was the only time in my school life when I got a spanking, and it was given by my mama, who was my teacher.

There was this boy who was in my grade at Blair's School. His name was Richard Bryant. The other students teased me about him being my boyfriend. Because of this teasing, I really did not like him at all.

This incident which led to a spanking took place on a snowy day. We were playing outside, and Richard and I got into a snowball fight. He got the best of me by blooding my nose. Both of us got a good spanking.

Mom did not do a lot of spanking, but she was not too good to lay one on a student.

Zona Royse, Columbia, October 4, 2008

Principal Disciplined by Mother

I remember that a principal disciplined a particular child, and the next morning the child's mother was there and boy, things got rough around there.

I was actually in that elementary school at that time and I remember what happened. She just about whipped that principal!

Most principals do a good job, but sometimes they make mistakes.

Bige R. Warren, Barbourville, November 20, 2008

Witnesses Required

When I taught school at Edmonton in the elementary school, I paddled quite a few kids. They were worse then, when you'd get them in the room all together. I paddled several.

Then it got to where you had to have a witness if you were going to paddle a child. We had to do that, but by the time you got a witness, you were out of the notion to spank the kid. If you were going to spank, they'd say, "Be sure you've got a witness." That was so they couldn't say you abused them.

Virginia Janes, Edmonton, September 22, 2008

Never Too Old for the Paddle

While I was teaching in high school I had a ninth-grade homeroom. My room was located down in the basement, as schools weren't as nice then as they are now. There were twenty-four boys in the ninth grade, and two or three of them were really mean. I would ask them to sit down, and one day early on in the year I said, "Now, boys, let me tell you something. You are going to sit down and be orderly so I can check the rolls."

I had only ten to twelve minutes to check the rolls, and we were mixed in homerooms. That's where the attendance came from, and it was really important that the teacher knew everybody [was] there.

I had this one boy that kept messing up. I said, "If you do that one more time, I'm going to bend you over this desk and spank you."

The other students didn't think I would do it. They didn't know him. Well, I had a paddle in a drawer because we did spank back then, and there was no problem. I guess he thought he would defy me, but I said, "You come on up to the desk just a minute."

He came up to the desk, and I just took him and twisted his back right down there and bent his tail right over that desk and gave him about seven or eight good licks. From then on I didn't have much trouble.

He was one of the only two boys I think I ever spanked.

Daphne H. Goodin, Barbourville, November 21, 2008

Empty Threat

When I was teaching at New Bethel in 1966, I spanked one of the boys. He came back to school the next morning and said, "My daddy is going to come up here on you."

I said, "Honey, let your daddy come. Bring him any time you want to."

Well, his daddy never did come, but I thought he was going to come to jump on me for what I did.

Laura Agnes Townsley Stacy, Barbourville, November 21, 2008

Bring Your Own Switch

I never did get spanked when I was a student in a one-room school, but some of the other kids did. And after I started teaching at one-room schools we didn't call it spanking like they do now. Back then we'd send the ones outside to cut a hickory switch when they needed to be punished. We'd use that instead of spanking them.

I don't think I ever had the girls to go get a hickory switch.

Bernice Shartzer, Caneyville, October 1, 2008

The Boss

The very first day of school, after we'd had the roll call and the traditional Bible reading, and whatever else, one old boy stood up in the back of the room and started to sing. I called him up front and said, "What's your problem?"

He said, "I decided to sing."

I said, "Bend over and take hold of your ankles and I think I can take that song idea out of your mind." I really tore him up with a paddle.

I think I paddled one or two others that day, and from then on the discipline problems were understood between the students and me.

That's the way things go. If you're not in control of things, I don't care what you do in life, you are a lost ball in high weeds.

My daddy had taught at that school about seven years. He said, "Noble, are you going to be the boss, or let the students be the boss?"

I said, "Pappy, you'll find out," and it wasn't long until he did find out.

Noble H. Midkiff, Whitesville, December 1, 2008

Preference for a Paddling

When I taught at Bruce School I put the names and marks on the board for disturbances caused by the students. These students had to stay inside the room for five minutes for each mark, or get one lick with a ping-pong paddle.

Usually, after five minutes they asked for their lick with the paddle so they could go outside and play.

Hale Murphy, Eddyville, December 31, 2008

The Threat Is Enough

Students at most rural schools were very reticent about talking to the "strange substitute" teacher, and I spent many a quiet day with students who would barely speak above a whisper. A schedule of lessons was usually always available and the students were very diligent about doing their assignments. The only time I came even close to having a discipline problem was at a school with four or five older boys.

One day when recess was over these boys decided they still wanted to cross a fence to gather hickory nuts. When I called them to come back they ignored me. I went back to the building, got the teacher's paddle, and proceeded to crawl through the fence.

They immediately turned around and came back, entered the building without a word, and the incident was never mentioned again.

Norma Ramsey Eversole, Mt. Vernon, January 5, 2009

EARL, ONE TOUGH CUSTOMER

Montgomery was the biggest one-room school in Logan County. I had fifty-four students, and I was eighteen years old. In 1936 there were forty-eight one-room schools in Logan County.

I knew that I had a tremendous job, and because of this I had to be sure I was a good disciplinarian. I had one boy in my school whose name was Earl Sadler, and I had been told by several people that he was impossible, so I was determined to conquer him if it were possible. The first week of school he was real sassy. I used a switch on him but you could only use a certain size switch.

One of the boys in his eighth-grade class came in, so I said to him, "Maurice, I want you to get a paddle and I'm going to wear him out."

Believe it or not, he came in with a big log! I said, "Go back and get a smaller switch." He did, and I finally made Earl pull his overalls up and I really switched him good. It wasn't too long after that when he gave me more trouble. It lasted about six weeks, so I thought, "What am I going to do with this boy?" I racked my brain. I said, "What in the world can I do to conquer that boy?"

Later on I wrote a book about my teaching years, and this bad boy Earl was living in Detroit. One Sunday I was in the kitchen just after my husband and I had just come home from church. My husband, George, was sitting out on the carport and said, "Oh, Helen, I don't know who this is." He was in a red Cadillac. "You've got a visitor."

I said, "My goodness, that's Earl Sadler." He came in and bought three of my books. He passed away about one year ago, and I went to his funeral.

Helen Raby, Elizabethtown, January 10, 2009

THE FURTHER ADVENTURES OF EARL

One day the boys were playing ball out behind the schoolhouse and they were throwing rocks covered with mud and hitting the school. The girls and I were out front jumping rope, but as soon as I heard the noise I went back there to see what was going on. Well, they were hitting the schoolhouse and making red spots on the white wall.

I stopped them from doing that.

Not many days passed until a second-grade boy, whose name was Ernie and who was so undernourished, was not chosen to be a member of the team. Earl said, "I'm not going to have him on my team. He will make an out."

I said, "Oh, yes, you are going to have him on your team."

He said, "I'm not going to do it, and I told you I'm not going to do it." He just kept arguing with me.

I said, "Okay, I'm going to expel you," and I did expel him. Then I said, "When you come back in three days—and don't you come back until those three days have expired—then bring your mama or daddy or somebody with you."

In three days he came back. When he was coming back, Maurice Hall, who was one of four eighth-grade students, said, "Miss Helen, don't say a word; I'll take care of him." Maurice took care of things, and he was just in the eighth grade. He really went to my defense.

I said to Earl's mother, "Let him tell you what's going on."

She said, "I didn't know he was doing all these things." Earl was born late in his dad's life and he just thought he could do whatever he wanted to do.

Earl's daddy said, "I'll fix that. I'm going to take you home and beat the devil out of you. I didn't realize you were doing that." So the problem was solved.

They were good people and they kept discipline on him. After that, we got along real well. I made a believer out of him.

Helen Raby, Elizabethtown, January 10, 2009

MOUTHER

I had one boy that was rebellious at times. I had to spank him, and he always showed a madness when I had to spank. This was when the teacher had control in the classroom, and when Daddy and Mama said, "If he disobeys, spank him."

That boy was a "mouther," but once I got control of him the spankings ceased.

Nell S. Eaton, Glasgow, January 8, 2009

Chapter 6

Daily Activities

Teachers in one-room schools were responsible for much more than teaching. The schoolhouse infrastructure was primitive, often without electricity or running water; teachers' chores ranged from lighting the stove in the morning (a responsibility sometimes delegated to a student for a small pecuniary consideration) to providing well water for drinking and washing to cleaning the schoolhouse to, on occasion, cooking the students' lunch.

Academic instruction itself was a much more complicated endeavor than it is today, as teachers were responsible for teaching eight grades of students—and this without the books and equipment that would nowadays be considered requisite. Academics focused on the basics, and it was common for teachers to rely on older children to help the younger ones, a practice many teachers believe had a positive educational value for all grades. Daily schedules followed a predictable format during school hours, 8:00 to 4:00, including morning recitation and seat work, though there were often special activities on Fridays.

There was plenty of time for play, however, with two daily recess periods. The stories below tell of favorite games, some of which will be familiar to today's children and some not, such as softball, marbles, red rover, and mumble peg. Lunchtime was also a popular part of the day. Children usually brought their lunch from home, typically homemade country food.

Typical Day at School

At the first school where I taught we had an opening program consisting of Bible readings and songs. For the first period, first graders were brought to a long recitation bench and were given instructions, then took turns reading aloud and spelling. After that they returned to their seats with purposeful seat work. The other classes followed.

At 10:00 a.m. we had a thirty-minute recess during which games were played. Then at 10:30 a.m. we began our arithmetic classes, and older students worked on yesterday's assignment. The younger ones were back to the recitation bench and given instructions and/or work on the blackboard, or flash cards.

Problems were written on the blackboard for them to write down and work on when they returned to their seats. The older students brought their work to be checked [and were] instructed about the new work and assignment until lunchtime at 12:00 noon.

We washed our hands with soap, and one person pouring water that had been carried from a spring. The water was poured with a dipper, and each child brought their water glass. After eating the children played games until 1:00 p.m.

When school began at that time, a story was read for "cool-down" time. This may be a continued book story, poem, or a short selection from Meriam Blanton Huber's *Story and Verse for Children*, published in New York. . . . In reading stories or reciting poems in unison, I'd sometimes stop to let them fill in the next word. . . .

Outside toilets were finally built, and an "In" and "Out" card was hung by the door to be used by the students.

Our recess in the afternoon lasted twenty to thirty minutes, then for the last period at school that day we studied geography, social studies, health, or history. School was dismissed at 4:00 p.m.

This pretty well sums the schedule and curriculum except for Friday afternoons. Sometimes we'd do special cleaning jobs, have a spelling contest, and do artwork.

Betty Holmes McClendon, Nancy, January 26, 2009

"All of Us Were Innocent"

At 8:00 a.m. each day we "took up books" by ringing a bell for roll call. At 8:10 we had a health inspection. The students lined up according to sex in two rows. I inspected their fingernails and their neck and ears for cleanliness. The hair of both boys and girls had to be combed so it would not fall into their eyes. Finally, the students opened their mouths to reveal whether their teeth had been brushed. None of the students objected to doing these things. I had learned the practice from my grandmother's stories.

I also taught the students that didn't own a toothbrush how to use a brush made from a birch twig, with the end pounded soft, dipped in baking soda to clean their teeth. Anyone failing the inspection received five demerits as part of the discipline system. They also received five demerits for getting on the floor if someone else was up, ten demerits for talking during class, ten for fighting, five for looking out the window—unless a car went by. When a car went by we all looked! When twenty-five demerits were accrued, the student was punished. They were removed each Friday.

The punishment for students in grades 1 through 4 was to memorize "The Village Blacksmith," and punishment for grades 5 through 8 was to memorize "The Raven." We called memorizing "learning by heart." Thankfully, very few of the students ever reached twenty-five demerits. . . .

After the health inspection we had devotionals. We said the pledge of allegiance and repeated the Lord's Prayer in unison. We took turns reading a chapter from the New Testament orally and sang "My Country 'Tis of Thee." After that we sang two or three more songs all together and with great gusto. Some of these songs were "The Papaw Patch," "John Brown Had a Little Indian," and "Froggie Went a-Courting."

By 8:30 we began our classes and worked steadily until recess. If a student needed a restroom break, they would look at the two cardboard signs hanging on each side of the door. One side said "In" and the other side said "Out," printed in red for the girls and blue for the boys. If a small child was gone too long, an older child would be sent to see about them. . . .

The last fifteen minutes of each day we read aloud a chapter from books like *Tom Sawyer* by Mark Twain, and *Taps for Private Tussie* by Jesse Stuart. These books were favorites of the children. Since no one was ever heard of in real life [with] a name like Tussie, the term "Lazy as the Tussies" became a favorite cliché when someone did not get their work, and in my youthful ignorance I did not reprimand them for saying it.

I would climb onto a chair and look in the mouth of a teenage boy approaching six foot tall to see if his teeth had been brushed. Yes, I was ignorant of what might have happened, but all of us were innocent. All these things happened forty-nine years and sixty years ago. Times have changed but not all for the better.

Betty Jo Arnett Lykins, Salyersville, February 9, 2009

Busy Day's Work

When I began teaching at a one-room school, things were the same as the school in which I had attended, except that we now had electricity. We had also learned a few new games. I was young and more active than my teachers had been, so I enjoyed playing games with my students.

When I began teaching the first year I had students from second grade through seventh grade, but no first- or eighth-grade students. I soon found out that students ranged from first to eighth grade in their learning ability.

I had a long chalkboard that reached from one side of the building to the other side, covering one end wall of the building. I kept one of the chalkboards covered with vocabulary words. I would have the first class's vocabulary drill, and one child could say the words, and if he or she knew them all, he could let the other children say them, one child at a time.

I could tell when they would miss a word by hesitating before saying the word. If it were the first child's turn and he/she didn't know all the words, they lost their turn as leader that day.

Since there were no spelling books for the first- or second-grade students, I made a book of words. I always put them on the board and the child copied them down after he/she learned to make the letters. I soon found that most of these students could make their letters and numbers, and could count when they came to school.

After the children had said their words, I would let them read orally, then put up new words for the next story.

I would give the first-grade class its lesson, then go on to the seventh-grade class. When their class was over and assignment or work given for the next day, they would go ahead and get their assignment, which included vocal words, etc. These older children would then be able to work with the first graders. Required readings would be over by 10 a.m. or 10:30 a.m., then came math exercise. After math came science, social studies, and health, with younger children learning from the older ones.

Some days we would be so busy that we would be a few minutes late getting out at the end of the day. . . . Parents thought children were playing on their way home.

Pauline Keene Looney, Pikeville, December 8, 2008

Conditions in a One-Room School

At the one-room school I attended, we had a round, potbelly stove and a hand-dug well. And we had only one outdoor toilet, used by both girls and boys.

The teacher would let the fire in the stove die down, then remove the ashes, put in paper, wood, and then put in lumps of coal if we had coal. One of the eighth-grade boys would come to school early to build the fire before other students got there. When the others got there, they would move their chairs as close to the stove as possible.

We had a hand-dug well at the back of the schoolhouse. To get water we used a zinc bucket with a rope and pulley. We had a dipper located in the water bucket, and we kept the bucket on the stage. We brought our own individual drinking glass from home. Some of the older boys would catch the teacher busy, then drink from the dipper while they kept an eye on the teacher. When that worked, they would provide a sly grin toward the other students.

We didn't have electricity in the schoolroom until I was in the eighth grade, and my brother and I had gone on to be a student in a consolidated school. Our school back then began in July, but when the consolidated schools began after Labor Day, my brother and I enrolled in the consolidated school in order to be better adjusted to a larger school. We found out that one-room schools were not behind in any subjects, but ahead in most.

Pauline Keene Looney, Pikeville, December 8, 2008

Daily Schooltime Activities

Back then we started school at 8:00, then at 10:00 we had a thirty-minute recess, then at 12:00 we had lunch. That afternoon we had about a fifteen-minute recess to give everybody a little break; then school was out at 4:00.

While the students were on recess, the older ones played ball, jump rope, hide and go seek, hopscotch, and things like that. The girls and boys all played together.

We drew water from a well with a bucket and a rope. That was always done by seventh- or eighth-grade boys. They all wore jeans and overalls, and we had a cooler inside the schoolhouse into which we poured the water. It had a faucet on it. Every child had to bring their own drinking cup. That's the way they got their water at school.

Of course, all students brought their own lunch. Most of the kids were primarily country kids, so most of them brought biscuits with sausage or jam on it, a piece of fruit, cookies, and things like that.

I didn't have any really poor kids, so all kids brought their own food. But sometimes they didn't have too much lunch, but they always brought something for lunch. None of the kids ever stole food out of the lunch boxes, or buckets, from other kids. But I do know there was one family that their daddy ran a grocery store, and he would bring goodies to school, but the kids would exchange those goodies for biscuits and ham.

Before lunch was eaten the students had to wash their hands. We used a wash pan for this purpose. Water was poured in the pan, and several students washed their hands in it with soap; then that water was poured out and clean water was put in the pan. I always let the little kids go first to wash their hands; then all the others washed theirs.

When kids went to the outhouses, I can't recall just what was used as toilet paper, but I suppose it was primarily Sears, Roebuck catalogs. At least they didn't use corncobs at school toilets!

Back then students did not go to another school to play it in a ball game. Games like that were played at home school on Friday afternoons, and many of the boys and girls played against each other. Sometimes even the teachers also played. I don't recall what part I played, but I would play with them! [*Laughter*]

Mayola Graves, Loretto, September 9, 2008

Daily Duties

As a teacher, I had to build the fires in the schoolhouse, and we found out that the milk cartons from our lunches made great kindling. We'd put our milk cups in the bottom of the potbelly stove, and then put in the kindling and the wood and coal.

I had lots of boys that volunteered to do that, and then we'd just light the fire at the bottom. I did not grow up around things like that, so building a fire was something I was not familiar with.

I also had big girls that volunteered to sweep in the afternoon.

Thus, I didn't have to do all the work myself, but I was responsible for everything. I also cooked the food on a two-burner hotplate. I would warm up a can of peas, and one delightful thing I thought was that we had some federal pork. I put tomato catsup in the pork and made barbeque sandwiches. They had a well-balanced meal.

The children in that community had gardens and plenty of food, but they didn't necessarily have a balanced meal. So I saw children grow inches, and their cheeks would get pink, and [they would] grow inches and gain pounds. They did well on the balanced meal. We always had bread, butter, milk, a vegetable, and meat. The county health person would plan the meals and tell the teachers how to prepare the meals.

They had some ragged clothes to some extent, but were clean. Overall, this was a pretty good community. They appreciated the teacher. Once I was helped by a neighbor, not a parent. On the main road, snow would not let me get over a small hill. The neighbor got some ashes and put [them] under my tire so I could get home.

I brought a record player to school, and the children loved it. A bag of candy was a treat to these appreciative students.

There was one TV in the neighborhood. The mother at that home came to school to tell about President Kennedy being shot.

Joyce Campbell Buchanan, Barbourville, November 21, 2008

LOG HOUSE ONE-ROOM SCHOOL

In 1935 I attended school in a one-room log schoolhouse which was approximately three-fourths mile from our house. My two older sisters and one older brother walked with me and held my hand as we walked across a footlog to get to school.

My fondest memories of that school was the times we could go outside and sit on a hand-hewn log bench for story time, and the tea set my teacher gave me as a Christmas gift was a blessing from heaven. It truly was a gift since we never had luxuries like that.

Half a year into my primer grade a new building was completed so we could go to a new cobblestone, two-room school, but we had to walk approximately two miles and a half to get there. Walking that far twice daily was a pretty good walk for a six-year-old.

Laura Agnes Townsley Stacy, Barbourville, November 21, 2008

Daily Bread

I started teaching in 1957 and was pregnant in 1964. Back then they had a law that you could not teach school if you were pregnant. So I took the year off, and my son was born in September. Once he was born, they called from the central office and asked me if I would substitute teach at Jeff's Creek one-room school where the teacher had been run off by the students. I went up there, and it was a poor sight when I got there. It was all dirty. I worked and cleaned everything up and had a hotplate to cook on then. I had to cook their lunch every day.

The county sent me canned green beans, turnip greens, butter beans, and some corn occasionally. They kids liked corn and would eat it. We never had any meat to eat.

All the kids were kind of shy then. When I met them, there were like four kids in one family, five in another. There were only seven or eight families that had kids in school there. I soon got really acquainted with all the families out there, and visited all of them to tell them about their children and talk about going on to high school.

When I first got there in October, we had only a water bucket, a dipper, and a big potbelly stove. I had to build a fire in the stove every morning to get the schoolhouse warmed up by the time the children got there.

I had several friends from Knox Central who had kids that had outgrown their clothes. All the children I taught were from very poor families, so I asked them one day, "What would you all like to have to eat?" I didn't wait around long either, so after two weeks I was down at the school board office asking them for meat for hamburgers. None had ever had one. I asked them at the office, "Where is the milk truck? We're supposed to have milk."

They told me that they used to get milk, but the truck could not get up there to the school. I said, "Well, we're going to get some milk again." I had it delivered to my house and carried it to school.

At home at night I made brownies, baked a cake, made homemade candy, cupcakes, and other treats for the children like canned peaches and a peach cobbler pie. These things I made would really delight them as they ate them.

I began making hamburgers, and soon got hotdogs for them. They absolutely loved it because they had not had anything else except green beans.

Daphne H. Goodin, Barbourville, November 21, 2008

Cool School

The hardest thing I had to deal with at school was in wintertime and having to get the school building warm in the morning. We had to build a fire, and the stove was always in the middle of the room. To get there in the morning the children would have to wear their coats and gloves, and keep their overshoes on until we got a fire built and the building warm. Of course, they wore warm clothing, such as long underwear, long stockings, and other things.

At Union Hill School, I had a little boy who was only in third grade, but he was an early bird! He liked to get there first and build a fire. He could get in because the building was never locked. I didn't even have a key to the building. Anyway, he would always come to build the fire for me.

When the kids got there, all of them wanted to sit around the stove, close to it. They wanted to be around the stove, because it was cold near the windows.

Betty Jane (Miller) Pence, Franklin, Tenn., September 29, 2008

Making the Rafters Ring

I attended Parnell School, a two-room school about a mile from home. One part of the building, called the "little room," housed first, second, and third grades. The other part, known as the "big room," housed the other five grades.

A very fond memory I have of my school was opening exercise each morning. First was Bible reading, then singing traditional songs like "My Old Kentucky Home," "Swanee River," "Carry Me Back to Old Virginny," and others. We would make the rafters ring!

Norma (Stephenson) (Coffey) Bertram, Monticello, March 5, 2009

Bible Readings

I remember we had Bible reading every morning, and I'm the one that did the reading most of the time. Back then we were free to pray if we wanted to. However, I think I depended on the Bible reading and didn't pray.

I didn't have any trouble from any of the children, because they all listened while I was reading.

Marguerite Wilson, Leitchfield, October 1, 2008

Spelling and Arithmetic Matches

Every Friday we'd have what we called a spelling match. Every Friday we had to do something, and if we didn't go play a ball game we'd have a spelling match. In the spelling matches, a kid on the opposite side would spell out a word, then the kid on the opposite side exactly across from him/her had to spell a word that began with the last letter in the word pointed out to them. Most of the kids tried to spell a word that ended with a "y" or an "x."

In the spelling contests they'd give out spelling words, and if the opposing student didn't spell the word correctly, they'd have to set down.

Sometimes we'd also have math matches, where the kids would go up to the board and divide up, then line up on opposite sides of the room. Then two of the kids would go up together, and you'd give out problems, and see which one got it first. The student that lost would have to sit down, then the next student went up to the board to enter the contest. They had lots of fun doing that.

The kids worked a lot to get ready for contest matches like that.

Virginia Janes, Edmonton, September 22, 2008

Ciphering Matches and Spelling Bees

Ciphering matches involved work with numbers. It began when students chose two team captains. These captains then took turns choosing numbers for their team. The names of the team captains were written on the blackboard located in front of the schoolroom, and the students' names were written under his or her name as they were chosen.

The lower-grade students were chosen first; thus the match started with students from first and second grades. One student from each team went to the blackboard and got his chalk and eraser.

The student chose the math area he/she wanted, then addition, subtraction, etc.

The teacher gave them a problem. Then the first one solving the question and giving the correct answer was the winner, and remained in that capacity to take on the next contestant.

This continued until one team's members were eliminated and the winner was the team that turned down the most members of the other team.

The spelling bee was a contest that was set up in the same manner as a ciphering match, with two teams contesting against each other. These spelling bees were based on words pronounced to each team by the teacher.

When a student failed to spell his or her word correctly, they were out of the game. The team that had the most members remaining at the end was the winner.

Virginia Galloway, Merry Oaks, December 3, 2008

Spelling Contests and Ball Games

Each week we would have a spelling elimination because so many of the students wanted to be in a spelling contest. As they missed spelling their words, they were out of the contest. It was certain school grades that participated in these spelling bees.

On pretty Friday afternoons, if the students all behaved well that week, we had a community ball game. A lot of the young people in the neighborhood that had already finished the eighth grade came and played ball with us. That was fun.

Mayola Graves, Loretto, September 9, 2008

School-Day Games

Back then these schools were in A-frame buildings. If the larger students could throw a ball over the building, they'd play ante over, and if you caught the ball over on the other side of the building, you ran around the building and tried to hit somebody with it. And if you hit them, they had to come over to your side of the building.

So that's how we'd break up the sides and win the game. The side that hit the most students won the game.

Another game we played was called hopscotch. We'd make a hopscotch yard by drawing it off. The girls really liked to play that game, but they didn't like to play marbles.

However, most of the boys wanted to play marbles. We called it "rolly hole marbles." It was played in a marble yard in which there were three marble holes. The kids would try to get there early in the morning so they could play a game before the bell rang to tell them that school was to start. The handbell I used was the same one my mother used, and I still have it.

What the girls liked most of all was to play jump rope.

In the wintertime, when students couldn't go outside to play, they'd play jacks. To do this, they'd clean the teacher's desk off in order to have a clean table on which to play jacks, which were ten little metal star-shaped things with a rubber ball. They'd toss the rubber ball to see how many jacks they could pick up before it bounces. You'd start by picking up one, then two, then three, and go all the way to ten. If you got to ten without messing up or dropping them, you won.

Another game we played was called tag. Usually you'd have two teams, and then just start running. And if you caught one of the other kids, they had to come to your side. Then they had to go ahead and try to catch someone of the other side. That's how you'd break up the sides. That was a game played by both boys and girls.

Softball games were very popular, and both boys and girls played that game. Other schools would sometimes come on Friday afternoons and bring their softball players to play us. That was especially true back when I was a student at Merryville School. Teams from other schools would just appear, and we didn't know they were coming. When that happened, our teacher would dismiss our classes, and we'd go out on the playground.

You can see that we had plenty of physical exercise.

Betty Jane (Miller) Pence, Franklin, Tenn., September 29, 2009

GAMES AND SOCIAL EVENTS

I, as did other one-room school teachers, held annual pie social events. The profits were used to buy educational materials. These events were well supported by the community. It was a social event anticipated by and attended by many persons.

Some of the favorite games were ante over, flying Dutchman, and of course, softball. Sometimes older girls would play games with the younger children. There was harmony; thus each was willing to share time with others. In mid-afternoon the students enjoyed a recess that lasted for fifteen minutes.

Patricia Gibson, Greenup, April 11, 2009

Fast-Racing Girls

My favorite memory of being a student in a one-room school was playtime. I could run fast. We would set up a base and see who could get there first.

As to whom I used to race against, it was most anybody that was running, but mainly boys. And yes, I did win.

I recall running against [the boy] who would eventually be my husband, Arnold, and also running against a long-legged boy. His name was Carl Corley, and he could run just about as fast as I did. Another competitor was Johnny Goodman.

All those boys were neighbors, of course. We were all good runners, but I beat them a lot of the time, even though I had short legs and they had long legs!

Bernice Shartzer, Caneyville, October 1, 2008

A Game Known as Indian

One of the big games kids in my one-room schools played was called Indian.

That was a game in which there were students that were Indians, and they would chase the others trying to catch them. They'd run from one tree to another tree, but if the Indians caught someone, that person had to get in jail. They would make a circle, and they all had to get in the circle.

Another way they played Indian was to put them on a base and they'd put their feet to where they'd have to touch the base and reach out as far as they could. Some of their friends could come and touch their hands before the Indians that was chasing them got them, and they'd get to go back home before the Indians got them.

I don't remember exactly how they played that game, but they did play it a lot. The ones that played in that game divided up, and then they decided who was going to be on which team.

Virginia Janes, Edmonton, September 22, 2008

GAMES PLAYED AT SCHOOL

In reference to the games children played, if it were raining, I had a checkerboard and they would play checkers on the inside. They also played fox and hound, and they played softball. The bat they used wasn't a bought bat; it was just a piece of wood that some kid brought from home.

We didn't have any competitions with other schools at that time.

The girls also played, and I played with them at times. I wasn't considered a coach, but I was there to oversee what went on.

The kids also played tag, and some of the smaller ones played drop the handkerchief, or something along that line.

Emma Walker, Eddyville, October 7, 2008

TEACHER PLAYS ALONG

My favorite game at school was called town ball. It was easily played and more suitable for the entire group of students to play. Another ball game was cap ball, a game in which every student threw their cap down in a circle and the leader would go around to pick up a ball that had been thrown over the house into somebody's cap. Then he would go around in a circle chasing the others in order to tag them. If he tagged someone, that person then had to go on the leader's side.

Then they'd go around in a circle chasing each other. The boys and girls all played that game, and I did also. That was my favorite game at school.

I also played on the softball teams with the students, and also played with them what was called ante over, drop the handkerchief, stink base, and other games such as mumble peg, which was played with a sharp-bladed knife.

When playing mumble peg, you would first lay the knife in the palm of your hand and make it go up into the air, then come down and sink [it] in the ground. If you did that okay, then you could go on and lay it on the back of your hand and flip it over and make it go in the ground. Before the game started, some of the kids would make a peg and hit it with their case knife and make the peg stick down in the dirt. When that was done, they'd give the player three times to hit the peg and try real hard to sink it into the ground. Then, in order to get the peg out of the ground, one of the kids had to bend down over the peg and try to pull it out with their teeth. That was somewhat of a dangerous game, especially when you had to flip your knife backwards over your head and make it stick in the ground.

The children made their own rules when playing those games, and you'd better follow their rules, or you'd probably lose it for the rest of your life!

Mamie Wright, Tompkinsville, October 16, 2008

Teacher Doesn't Play

The games schoolkids played back then included red rover; duck, duck, goose; handkerchief; and baseball. They played a lot of baseball. When playing the duck, duck, goose game, the kids sat in a circle and [one] would go around saying, "Duck, duck goose." It's probably the same thing as playing handkerchief, a game in which they'd have to get up and chase them to see whoever gets back first.

All kids, both boys and girls, liked to play ball, either baseball or softball, depending on whatever kind of ball they had. We didn't play other school teams, just played each other.

I never could hit the ball, so they never wanted me to play! I think I just sat on the sidelines and would yell and everything, to cheer them on.

Maryanna Barnes, Frankfort, October 14, 2008

Pretty Girl Station

We had no toys at school except for a plow line or rope which were used for the game jumping rope. We also had a long flat board with a hole in each end. The rope was used to make swings over the limb of a tree.

We played fox and dog and pretty girl station. In the latter game, we chose players for two teams. One team would march toward the other team's line. We would say to the other team, "We are from pretty girl station."

Members of the other team would say, "What is your occupation?"

The first team would then say, "Almost anything."

The waiting team would then say, "Get to work on it, then."

The visiting team would have already decided what they would be doing before marching to meet the other team [and the children would pantomime performing an activity]. For example, if the answer was "Washing clothes" and it was guessed, then the visiting team would run back to their home base. However, those who were caught had to go home with the other team.

At the end of the fifteen-minute recess, the team with the most players won the game.

Pauline Keene Looney, Pikeville, December 8, 2008

TWIRLED MARBLES

At school, if one kid starts picking on another one, it was probably settled somewhere out of school by riding on little scrapling bushes. Back then they would cut the little bush, then bend it over and get on it to have the best rides.

Another game they played at Rock Bridge was called marbles. The kids used to take their homemade stone marbles over to Audie Irvin's spring, where the water flowed down from a low strip of flat stone. They would put their marbles in a stone container, place it under the waterfall so that the water could twirl the marbles around and around until they got slick and round. I seem to recall that the twirling took about two weeks to get the job done.

Some of the kids went ahead and used glass marbles when playing the game, but these stone marbles would split the glass marbles in two.

Some of the kids got to school early just to be able to play marbles before school started. Wallace McGuire, Charles and Lynwood Montell, and several others always did that. I always think of Wallace and Charles and Lynwood as playmates.

Mamie Wright, Tompkinsville, October 16, 2008

CRACK THE WHIP

We used to play a game called crack the whip. It was really a rough game because we got a big line of children to hold hands. We always got the bigger boys up front, and they would start running and swinging the other children around and try to whip the other one off that was the farthest away on the end. And when they whipped them off, they would just throw them anywhere.

I don't know how we really kept from getting some of them hurt really badly, but we never did hurt them that way. But they were hurt a little bit, such as being rolled around and bruised up, but not hurt too badly.

Wanda Humble, Monticello, November 7, 2008

Fox and Hounds

Most of the schools I taught were in the edge of the woods, and one of the games we played was called fox and the hounds. Some kids would be the hounds and others the foxes. The hounds would chase the foxes. We'd run out into the woods and hide on the big rocks.

Those kids would have a hard time catching me because I could outrun most of them!

Alma New, Monticello, November 7, 2008

Rough Game

The bigger kids played a game we called rabbit. You would catch a person and hold them until a hunter could shoot them with a soft rubber ball. I played that game with them, and I'd get caught so that I could catch others. And I'd just wait until one of the big boys came around the circle just as fast as he could come. When he'd come by, I would hit him right in the stomach with all the power in my shoulder. Then he'd hit me!

During school I'd put my hands on his shoulder and say, "Do I need to talk to you about this?" He would shake his head to say no.

I punished him on the school ground in the name of the game. I knocked the breath out of him because I knew the idea of waiting until the last moment to hit him full speed in the stomach with my shoulder. I just flattened him!

I didn't have to spank him because he knew I could. I'd pick him up and say, "Are you hurt? Are you hurt?"

He didn't say anything at first because he had the breath knocked out of him. When you have the breath knocked out of you, you think you are licked; you think you are dying. [*Laughter*]

Irma Gall, Barbourville, November 20, 2008

Beating the High Schoolers

In July 1942 I was assigned to teach at the Hamilton School, but taught there only three months before Uncle Sam gave me a notice to report for duty in the military during World War II.

During that first three months at Hamilton School, we had a good enrollment of forty to fifty children. We had a bunch of larger boys, and we had a good softball team. Softball was a major sport with the larger kids, and we were so good that we challenged Summer Shade High School, located in southern Metcalfe County, to a softball game.

I took the boys to Summer Shade one afternoon and played them in softball. Well, they defeated us by a small score, but on the next Friday the Summer Shade High School team came to Hamilton and returned the game to us. We defeated them there at Hamilton.

That was sort of a landmark. The Hamilton students thought that was real great to defeat a high school team! Our team was really good. I was their pitcher, and I had a big tall boy on first base. Each space was filled with good players. The players in the field backed me up. They'd catch those fly balls and tag the opposing players out at first base.

That game was something I remember very distinctly.

J. Robert Miller, Rock Bridge, September 18, 2008

Beating the High Schoolers Again

At Big Creek I had a basketball team. The teacher that was there before me was a man, and he really worked with them in basketball. When I was teaching there, we were invited to some other places to play the schools there. So I went on and tried to coach that basketball team. My husband helped me some, but I took my team to Adair County High School and played them and won the game. Can you imagine? We were a one-room school and we beat the high school team. We had some good players.

Then I came over to Edmonton where my brother-in-law was teaching, and coaching a team. We also beat them.

I taught at two other one-room schools, but I guess Big Creek was my favorite school.

One of the other schools at which I taught was Angely. We played a lot of baseball. I'd load my car up with those kids. And we'd go to other schools on Friday and play them. We all rode in my vehicle, unless there were some parents that wanted to go, but I didn't have too many that went.

I played with my team, and one teacher at the other school didn't like it. She said she didn't think teachers were supposed to play on the team. I said, "Well, I have to play because I won't have enough players. You have to have nine."

One of the things I remember about an injury at this school is that I stumped my toe and fell on second base. It was real dusty, and dust just flew. And the players got just as quiet as a mouse until I got up and sort of laughed, then they just wahawed!

They were afraid I was hurt, but I said: "I'm alright."

When I said that they all started laughing and said, "Boy, you made the dust fly!"

Virginia Janes, Edmonton, September 22, 2008

MASTERFUL STORYTELLER

On Friday after the last recess the teacher would ask if someone wanted to tell a story: a story from a book or just a story. We had one boy that would just get up and tell stories that fascinated all of us children. This could be about something like going bear hunting or fishing.

To do this, he would just go on and on with his story, making up things at times as he continued. He had a vivid imagination and we were held spellbound when he told his stories.

Pauline Keene Looney, Pikeville, December 8, 2008

MAPPING FUN

We made a big thing out of Halloween, which was all meanness. Christmas was a big event; then usually on Valentine's Day we would sponsor moneymaking things so we could take a school trip going around Stinking Creek to see where all the schools were. We would visit them to play ball at one school, play ball at another, eat lunch at another. That was a big deal!

They could draw free hand. Anybody at the first of the month could go to the board and draw free hand a whole map of Stinking Creek and put on all the schools, churches, and post offices.

They knew the location of each school because every day I would go to the board and draw them; then the students would draw them and put even more things in the map.

Irma Gall, Barbourville, November 20, 2008

ALL IS WELL

I was with my schoolchildren during lunch and recess, so there was never a fight at my school. There were no lunch boxes at lunch time, only paper bags that consisted mostly of biscuit snacks brought from the homes. The children never seemed to be lacking in nutrition.

They all said they had a hot meal in the morning before school and in the evening after school at home. I never had a complaint about one student stealing from another, and the students were respectful of each other.

Stella K. Marcum, Pikeville, February 10, 2009

EAGER FOR LUNCHTIME

The morning session was broken with a fifteen-minute recess for fun and exercise. Then at lunchtime the contents of tin buckets, or a few so-called lunch boxes, were opened. Some kids brought biscuits with sausage, or biscuits and jelly. A few would bring peanut butter and crackers. Some would have purchased snacks from May Webster's store on the way to school.

Everyone was in a hurry to finish lunch so the rest of the time could be spent in play.

Patricia Gibson, Greenup, April 11, 2009

FRIED GREEN TOMATOES

Kids brought their lunches to school in lunch buckets. Some of them used lard buckets; some of them used nice, pretty lunch buckets. I remember one day when a boy came around to me, and he was eating a biscuit sandwich. He said to me, "Mr. Robert, do you know what that is?"

I said, "No, what is that?"

He said, "That's fried green tomatoes. I've got four of them in my lunch bucket."

He was really proud of those fried green tomatoes. Today we consider that a delicacy.

Of course, the kids brought with them sausage and biscuits, ham and biscuits, fried pies, baked sweet potatoes, tomatoes, apples, fried chicken, and other things such as butter beans and peas in cans. Some brothers and sisters brought separate lunch buckets, but others would jointly share the basket, or larger bucket.

That was a family situation, just whatever they chose to do.

J. Robert Miller, Rock Bridge, September 18, 2008

School Lunch

While teaching at one-room schools, my lunch usually consisted of a scrambled egg sandwich that I fixed that morning at home. I would also have an apple, an orange, or some other type of fruit. I also loved peanut butter sandwiches, just as the kids did. I took those sandwiches in a dinner bucket when I was a child in school. I still have my dinner bucket I used back then.

When the federal lunch program came into being in the early sixties, teachers just ate with the kids. Peanut butter was so very popular and appreciated back then.

We had good healthy food, such as milk, cheese, peanut butter, and beef. We would warm up the food on the potbelly stove and enjoy a good meal.

The girls did most of the cooking.

Bige R. Warren, Barbourville, November 20, 2008

Lunch from Home

When I was teaching at Bee Spring Elementary School, the old road, which was dirt, was very close to the new road. Students would walk to school on the dirt road, and some would take a short cut across the hollow.

I had one student that had polio early in life and she would ride a horse to school.

Students would bring milk in a jar and set it outside on the concrete well to get it cold. If it froze out there, they would lick the frozen ice. For food, they brought from home eggs between a biscuit. In the winter they would have hog meat and bacon. They also had some kind of fruit for dessert.

The poor students walked home for lunch, but sometimes there was nothing for them to eat when they got there. To my knowledge, no food was ever stolen.

Michael M. Meredith, Bee Spring, December 7, 2008

CORNCOB FIGHTS

In the summer everybody had gardens, so the students' lunch boxes reflected what was in the garden. There would always be fresh tomatoes, corn on the cob, jelly biscuits, and fried green tomatoes on a biscuit. But in the wintertime their food items would revert to peanut butter and crackers, homemade muffins, and whatever meat was left over at home, such as biscuit with sausage on it, tenderloin, cookies, and other things.

I don't remember any food theft that took place, but I remember the kids swapped food, especially brothers and sisters.

In the summertime we'd go outside and sit under the trees and eat lunch. Each one had their own lunch pail, and they'd have corn on the cob. When they had finished their corn on the cob, they would have corncob fights. When they did this they would call each other pigs. They would say, "Oink, oink," then throw these corncobs to hit another student! Then the student that got hit would throw a cob back to hit somebody on the other side.

Betty Jane (Miller) Pence, Franklin, Tenn., September 29, 2008

SUPERINTENDENT LOVED TO EAT

I was teaching at Rolly Creek. It was wintertime. We had windows on every side of the building. I looked out the window and saw the superintendent, Mr. Bell, coming to our school. He wasn't driving, as there was no way to drive to the building. He was walking in through the schoolyard, and we were all eating lunch.

He came into the building. He loved to eat. That day I shared part of my lunch with him. He stayed for just a few minutes, then left.

Imogene Dick, Monticello, November 7, 2008

LUNCH FOODS

Most of the children at Walnut Hill School had reasonably good food.

They would bring biscuits, jelly, peanut butter and crackers, fruit in season, and sometimes cake and pie.

The poorer kids had more breads, jellies, and strictly homegrown foods. Thankfully, I do not recall any stealing of food by those kids.

Some of the kids in school that year lived close enough to school that they could go home for lunch.

Nell S. Eaton, Glasgow, January 8, 2009

THROWING LUNCH

The kids would bring pretty good food, such as biscuit and sausage, biscuit and ham, fried pies, and things like that. Some of them would bring baked potatoes and sweet potatoes.

All of the kids brought their own lunch food. I don't remember any of them that couldn't bring anything to eat. But I do seem to remember that some of the kids did steal food from other buckets every now and then. Sometimes it was brothers and sisters that would get into each other's boxes. And they would get into a fuss when that happened.

I remember when I was going to school there at Penick, and people got to laughing at my sister next to me, and that caused her to begin throwing her lunch. They'd laugh, and she'd throw it until her whole lunch was thrown away.

There were three of us sisters, and me and the other one had to share food with her.

We had some good times at those rural schools.

Virginia Janes, Edmonton, September 22, 2008

COOKING AT SCHOOL

We got some commodities for Hebron School, as they brought commodities to the schools. I thought, "Well, how in the world am I going to cook rice, raisins, and pinto beans?" Well, I brought a big kettle from home. Of course, the children brought their lunches in paper sacks, a lunch bucket, a lard bucket, or whatever. So I kinda supplemented their cold food, which usually consisted of maybe sausage and biscuit, bacon and biscuit, or even bologna and biscuit, things that were left from breakfast; or a baked sweet potato, fruit of whatever kind was in season.

Back to my cooking experience, which took place on a large coal-burning stove located in the center of the room. I cooked rice, and they'd say, "Well, we're tired of it like this."

I said, "Well, did you ever eat rice with raisins cooked in it?"

No, they never had that. I said, "Well, alright, we're going to have rice and raisins today." I'd go ahead and cook a big pot, and they liked it. I also had each one of them to bring their own bowl and spoon from home. Back then we didn't have plastic spoons and throwaway utensils like we have today.

So I fixed a place in the cloakroom and put everybody's name up there, and they could put their bowl and things up there. Of course, it wasn't very sanitary as far as disinfectants were concerned, but we did wash the bowls and spoons and put them back up there clean.

And they did enjoy eating pinto beans, so I thought I'd also make some cornbread. I'd say, "We'll just fix some pinto beans and cornbread and have that today." The kids really did enjoy eating that.

I got some of the older girls to help me in preparing this, and they took part in it. So those were pretty good times, and at least none of them starved. And I don't remember having any overweight children like we have in schools today.

Emma Walker, Eddyville, October 7, 2008

TEACHER DELIVERED AND COOKED FOOD

At Allens Creek, I think I had eighteen students, had forty-two at Brotton, and sixty at Shady. There at Shady there was not enough room for all students to sit down at one time. We gathered around the table and at the board. I think one of the hardest things I did is when we were put up on the milk program. I could take [it] because I just gave milk to the students. That was during the 1960s. Every child was entitled to one cup of milk each day. Can you imagine how you were going to get milk to that school?

A lot of teachers refused to do it, so I got up early and delivered milk from a store on Stinking Creek to all these one-room schools before I started teaching that day. I drove a jeep when I did that.

In 1963 or '64, we had to have a hot lunch program. I had sixty kids, and actually had a little apartment by the school. Otherwise, I got one or two hotplates in order to serve hot meals to all my kids in that classroom, where we didn't have running water or anything.

At some schools, as fast as the food was delivered, the next day it wasn't there. Somebody was stealing it, especially this one little boy. The ones that stole food only stole what they wanted to eat. The mustard greens were the only things left. Peanut butter, pinto beans, and the number 10 cans of peaches were going very fast.

As soon as the food was delivered, we really had a feast. It was all free food for the kids, but all during my school time, I had to prepare that lunch.

I soon realized that other teachers in the community paid someone else to come and cook for them, but I didn't do that.

Irma Gall, Barbourville, November 20, 2008

"Right Cozy Place" for Lunch

Children brought lunches to school, usually in lard buckets, so called because stores sold lard in half-gallon buckets. They made nice lunch pails, having tight-fitting lids, and mothers would use nails to make little holes in them in order to help the air circulate. If there were several children in one family, gallon buckets would be used.

Biscuits with blackberry jelly or apple butter were standard lunch-time fare. Wild blackberries were plentiful and resourceful mothers picked them and made jam and jelly. The jelly would soak into the biscuits and make them a pretty purple. Even now when I wear purple, I think of those beautiful purple biscuits. Fried egg sandwiches would have made a nourishing change, but mothers saved eggs to take to the store and trade them for sugar, coffee, and flour, things that could not be grown on the family farm.

Some children brought milk with cornbread crumbled in it. That was standard menu for supper; the evening meal was never called dinner. Children also brought fried potatoes on biscuits, or on cornbread at times. A few would sometimes bring sausage or bacon. One little boy brought his milk to school in a whiskey bottle!

There was no designated place to eat lunches. Some ate under our big shade tree; some inside the schoolhouse, and some *under* the schoolhouse. Our yard was sloping and one end of our building had concrete blocks for a foundation. There was no underpinning, so some children liked to crawl under the house and eat lunch. It was a right cozy place. At times I would crawl under the house and sit cross-legged to eat with them.

Usually, I did circulate among the children as I ate my sandwich.

Vera Virgin, Greenup, January 21, 2009

Food Thieves

At Oak Hill we had a classroom and another small room that was called a vestibule. It had shelves on which the kids placed their lunch containers. Sometimes a hungry kid would go out there when I'd be busy. He would steal something to eat out of somebody else's lunch bucket.

That wasn't a major problem, but it did happen. When I found out what had taken place, I criticized him. Since he was hungry, I didn't consider it a bad crime for him to do that, but it was something he shouldn't do. I'd say, "You shouldn't do that. This lunch belongs to another person."

Usually, it would be a poor kid that did that because he didn't have enough to eat, so he would do a little mooching from some of the other kids. You could expect that.

J. Robert Miller, Rock Bridge, September 18, 2008

Stolen Pie

I got to school by 8:00 in the morning, and stayed until 4:00 in the afternoon. We had a fifteen-minute recess at 10:00; then we had an hour for lunch, because everybody brought their lunch and had to sit down and eat.

The food they brought for lunch was whatever they had at home, like fried potatoes, fried eggs, and some meat if they had it. They all had butter and sugar in a biscuit. Some of them brought molasses and/or syrup in a little jar.

On one occasion one little boy saw another boy's fancy custard pie that this boy's mother had cooked for him. He had a beautiful slice, and I can see it now. Well, I saw this one boy eating the other boy's pie.

The Stinson schoolhouse was high off the ground, and he was up under the floor eating that pie!

I scolded him, but can't remember whether or not I spanked him.

Bernice Shartzer, Caneyville, October 1, 2008

Taking a Dip

Something that was a problem was the unavailability of drinking water. At Merryville School, two students would walk across the road to Frank Miller's well. They took with them a metal bucket with a dipper in it and they would pump the bucket full of water and carry it back to the school. That was our drinking water that would sometimes last all day. We all drank out of the same dipper, unless you had your own drinking cup.

When one of the kids took a dipper of drinking water, if they didn't drink it all, they'd toss it out the door, then put the dipper back into the bucket. And even if they drank it all from the cup, they'd stick the dipper back into the bucket.

At Bowman and Union Hill schools, there was no water well close, and I'm not really sure, but I don't think we had any drinking water, except what they brought with them. Both schools were in faraway areas, not close to houses.

Betty Jane (Miller) Pence, Franklin, Tenn., September 29, 2008

Water Ways

Sometimes we got water for drinking purposes from a bored well over at a house. To be excused from school to go draw and get the water was a big deal. It was the bigger boys that went there to get the water.

The Stinson School had a bored well on school grounds. A bored well was made by using machinery to bore a hole in the ground, and case it. Then you had a bucket that you sent down into the well to draw the water out.

A dug well was dug by hand and lined with stones. And you had a well box over it, and a pulley that was used to send the bucket down and draw up the water. The county paid for the cost of providing wells for water. Some schools had bored wells and some of them had dug wells. Others got water from a spring.

There was a shelf near the door for the water bucket and dipper. Each child brought his/her own drinking cup and stored it on the shelf. They did *not* drink from a common cup, nor from the dipper.

Bernice Shartzer, Caneyville, October 1, 2008

MAKING DO

When I went to a one-room school, we took for our lunch at school just whatever Mama had cooked. Things like corn on the cob, an egg sandwich, or whatever, is what we took from home.

And also back then we didn't have a pencil sharpener or anything. Some of the boys brought knives, so we would line up every morning and sharpen pencils for everybody at school.

We'd also take our own drinking cups, as that was before the days of plastic. Usually the cups we used were something like empty vegetable cans. Everybody would line up in front of the water bucket to get their cups of water.

I learned how to make paper cups out of used paper. We'd use paper cups for water if we didn't have a can.

So, that's sort of the way it was when I attended a one-room school.

Zona Royse, Columbia, October 4, 2008

DUSTPANS NOT INCLUDED

At the beginning of the school year when I first started teaching, teachers and students would meet on Saturdays before school started. It was pretty much an all-day affair, and you didn't get paid for it, but you had to go.

At the end of the day the county would give you a dipper, a galvanized two-and-one-half gallon bucket, a box of chalk, two erasers, and a broom, but no dustpan. If you wanted a dustpan you had to furnish your own. We also got an order for five gallons of floor oil, because the floors were wooden and would get dusty, so we had to oil the floor. Those were the supplies we got, but no money to buy anything else.

We had to carry water to the schoolhouse. Many of the wells were not there at the school, so students would carry the water; then we would sterilize it by putting something like ten drops of bleach in a bucket of water. That was another one of the rules we had to follow.

Some schools did have water wells on the premise, and we carried water from neighbors.

Zona Royse, Columbia, October 4, 2008

Bugles and Buckets

The one-room school I attended was Steep Hollow around 1913, and Miss Gertie Lindsey was my first teacher. I forget how many years I went there to school, but we did walk to Brownsville after that. We had to cross Green River in a ferry. That was where I finished the other grades, except for one year in Indiana, where my father had a quick job.

Steep Hollow is about four miles from Brownsville, and that's what I walked each day; eight miles total. But when I went to Steep Hollow, I lived only about one-quarter of a mile from school. And we had an old man that lived on the way home, and he could play a bugle. Every afternoon at school, he would be setting out under a tree waiting for the schoolchildren to come so he could blow his bugle for them as we passed by.

There were quite a few kids in school there. Miss Gertie taught all eight grades, so our schoolhouse was pretty well full.

To get water, we'd go to a spring to get it, as we didn't have water any other way. We got the water in buckets. The kids that went to get the water had to walk down a little hill; then there was a water spring under that hill. They had a bucket that went down to the water on a rope, then the boys pulled it back up. You could walk down to the spring, but you couldn't carry the buckets full of water back up the hill very well.

Two boys did that job each time, and they were older than the younger kids, thus were stronger.

We drank the water out of a dipper, but we soon learned to bring our own cup. We did that all the years that I went to school there.

Blanche Demunbrun, Glasgow, September 30, 2008

Homework at School

The students at Fairview all had long walks to get to and from school, varying from two to three miles. I walked home with some of the students and, believe me, it was a long walk through the woods and across the ridges. It was even further when it rained or snowed. Even though the kids arrived home late, they still had chores to perform, thus did not have time for school homework. Additionally, if they did not have older siblings, there generally would be very little assistance available to help with the homework.

I was fresh out of school and knew the drudgery of homework. My solution to the problem was to make time available during the school day for them to do their homework. That way it was sure to be done and done right. A classmate, older student, or I could help as needed. The kids were bright enough to keep up, even when they had to miss school to work at home during the tobacco season, or for other crop plantings/harvestings.

William H. Nicholls Jr., The Villages, Fla., December 14, 2008

Chapter 7

Outhouses

One-room schoolhouses did not have indoor plumbing. Most schools had outhouses—one for the girls and one for the boys—though in some cases the "outhouse" was simply the great outdoors. Aside from their usual purpose, outhouses, as a few stories below illustrate, played a particularly satisfying role on Halloween.

His and Hers

Peddler Gap School had two outhouses out back. They were state-of-the-art facilities at that time, with moons and a star cut in each side and outdated catalogs for use as toilet paper.

These outhouses, or privies, were marked "His" and "Hers," and each building was equipped with two seats, [one with] a small hole cut for smaller children, and [one with] a large hole cut for larger students.

If students didn't have a problem with modesty, two students could use these facilities at the same time.

Jimmie Jones, West Liberty, December 29, 2008

The Boys' Book Policy

I remember what the policy was when you went to the outhouse. The girls had an outhouse but the boys didn't have one. We went down into the woods and got behind a tree. But when you left the classroom you were supposed to lay a book in the door. I remember that when the bigger boys would go out, they'd slam that book down and make a lot of noise, then they'd go on down behind a tree. When they came back they'd pick up the book. That way you knew someone [had returned from being out].

I don't remember whether the girls did a book in the door or not, but that was the policy the boys used.

J. Robert Miller, Rock Bridge, September 18, 2008

Very Unsanitary

One of the neighbors that lived close to the schoolhouse had to pass by the boys' toilet when going to get a bucket of water and taking it back to her house. The big old eighth graders knew about what time she'd come through there. And in those outdoor toilets you had about one and one-half foot of space at the top between the roof and the walls.

About the time she got through there, these boys would urinate through that hole into her water bucket. When that happened, she'd go straight up to the teacher and say, "They've done it again!" [*Laughter*]

The teacher always wore them out—I mean, wore them out!

Those outdoor toilets were a disgrace; they were awful. They were never cleaned, even though students used the seat, the floor, and everything, when they went to the toilet. Even bees were always flying and crawling around there, and it was just terrible.

When doing number two, you never sat on the lid, just squatted down since you were afraid to sit down because there was urine and feces everywhere.

Pat McDonald, Barbourville, November 21, 2008

Outhouse Accident

This is a story about what could have been a fatal accident. A little first grader went to the privy or outhouse. We had a note up under the boys' and girls' signs that said "In" and "Out."

When he went to the privy he was gone a little longer than usual and I was busy. His brother Gene, in the third grade, noticed that his brother was still gone. He came up to me and said, "Mr. Noble, Norman hasn't come back."

I said, "Go down there and check on him."

He went out there, then came running back and whispered in my ear and said, "Norman is in there."

I rushed down there, jerked my shirt off, and threw my arm down in there. He grabbed my hand just like a set of clamps, and I snaked him out. Well, he was standing in that gook up to his chin.

That actually happened and could have been a real tragedy.

When I got washed up and went back into the classroom, all the students were sitting around and talking. I told them, "I do not want this to be brought up tomorrow, or any other day, about Norman's bad luck."

They never did mention it after that.

Noble H. Midkiff, Whitesville, September 1, 2008

Before Outhouses

I went to a one-room school, but thankfully we had boys' and girls' toilets. However, I've heard stories that the older schools where my dad went and also where my mom went, that they truly just used the woods. Evidently they didn't have an outside toilet. They went down behind a tree, or over the hill where they couldn't be seen.

Bige R. Warren, Barbourville, November 20, 2008

Nature's Outhouses, Part 1

When I taught at Rolly Creek School we didn't have an outhouse. The school was located at the edge of the woods, and there was a path that went one way and a path that went another way. The boys went on one path, and the girls went the other, and they'd go out their path far enough to not be in sight of the school. I guess they went behind a big tree and used that as an outhouse. I guess the kids used tree leaves as toilet paper.

That was also true for me as well, as I had to walk along the girls' path when I needed to go.

Alma New, Monticello, November 7, 2008

Nature's Outhouses, Part 2

I taught at Rolly Creek School, and I remember quite well having to walk down a path from the school to the woods in order to have a place where number one and number two could be done. That was hill country, and when you went out you could get behind a hill. That's what I always did so nobody could see me!

I guess I always had paper tissues that I took with me to use after doing number two, but I don't remember what the children used. After we got outdoor toilets, we would use a Sears, Roebuck catalog.

I don't ever remember any boys or girls slipping up on each other when they were outside doing what they had to do. Boys and girls didn't go outside at the same time. There was an "In" and "Out" sign on the school door that the person had to display when they went out.

Imogene Dick, Monticello, November 7, 2008

Toilet Turning

We [the boys] had an outdoor toilet and the girls had one. We had little cards hanging on the wall on a string. Students going to the outdoor toilet flipped the card to say "Out" or "In." Well, some of us got the bright idea to turn them a time or two, and there would be three or four of us out.

One day when some of us were out, the teacher came down there and said, "What are you having, a party?" Then he whipped us all the way up the hill with a big switch!

Every Halloween the older boys would turn over both of the outdoor toilets, and the county workers would have to come and set them back up. That was a whole lot of toilets to set back up because kids did it all over the county. I think we had eighty-five one-room schools at one time before they started consolidating them.

But I never did turn the toilets over!

Pat McDonald, Barbourville, November 21, 2008

Tip or Treat

When I was going to a one-room school it was typical for older kids to play pranks during Halloween, such as turning outhouses upside down. I recall that happening two or three times where I went to school. I probably helped to do it, or was at least aware that it was going to take place.

The outhouses would be turned over so everyone could see the next day what had happened. Of course, the teacher would recruit a couple of neighbors to come and set the outhouses back up.

Bige R. Warren, Barbourville, November 20, 2008

Chapter 8

Getting to and from School

Traveling to and from school could be quite an adventure, sometimes even dangerous. Rural schoolhouses were typically in remote areas, and teachers and students alike often had to travel miles to reach them, frequently along muddy roads or across swollen creeks. Feet, mules, horses, cars, and the helpful arms or backs of other people served as means of transportation in the stories that follow.

Air-conditioned Jenny

This has to do with the time when I attended the Merryville rural [one-room] school. I started as a student there in 1925 and 1926. My brother and I went to Merryville School, and our sister Betty Jane did too.

When I was in the third or fourth grade, my dad decided that we ought to ride to school, so he bought a jenny from Raymond Bray for five dollars! A jenny is a female donkey, and we'd put a big saddle on that jenny. My dad would catch that jenny of a morning, put the saddle on it, then we'd get up in that saddle and ride the jenny to school.

That jenny had three rates. It was slow, slower, and slowest. [*Laughter*] You could whip it with a stick, but it wouldn't go any faster. It had big ears that flopped and a long tail. We were the only kids that had free transportation to school at that. Another thing I'd like to point out is that that transportation was air-conditioned! [Laughter]

I'll never forget that. But we grew up and got to the point that we wouldn't help take care of that jenny, so our daddy sold it for $7.50. He made some profit on it and that helped get our education.

J. Robert Miller, Rock Bridge, September 18, 2008

Helpful, Caring Brothers

When I went to Hamilton School I had four brothers but no sister, so my brothers looked after me on the way to school. When we got to the little stream that crossed the road, it would get muddy on some days. My brothers would put on their hip boots and carry me across the stream on their backs.

Mamie Wright, Tompkinsville, October 16, 2008

Musical Mule

When it rained a lot one low place in the road got flooded. Once the water got so high that our neighbor was generous enough to carry us across the water on his mule. He would place as many of us on the old mule's back as there was room for.

Of course, the old mule was so heavily loaded he "played music" [with his bowels] as he moped along.

Laura Agnes Townsley Stacy, Barbourville, November 21, 2008

Teacher's Travels and Travails

The first year I taught at Gregory, my brother was in the eighth grade there, along with an eighth-grade boy who was my neighbor. Well, he had a bicycle, and my other brother also had a bicycle, so we rode a bicycle two and one-half miles to school.

One day it had rained, and we lived on this country road. The water was standing on the road in ditches. On our way home, I was riding on the bicycle behind my brother, as I didn't ride my bicycle at that time. Well, the bike scooted off the road, and we fell on our backs right over into a mud hole!

I walked the rest of the time, but when I started teaching at Big Sinking School, my husband got me an old truck. . . . The road up there was bad, jumpy, and rocky. I got up there alright by jumping the truck up and down over rocks.

One of my neighbors went to school up there, and he rode with me up there and back. Well, one day it came a big rain; rained just about all day. I never thought about Big Sinking Creek getting up high, so we got back down there to the creek to cross it. But before we got there, we saw this big board laying out on the road, and we stopped and got out to see what it was. Well, it was a board that had nails all in it. We went on down to cross the creek, and it was up high and really muddy. It looked terrible, so I didn't know whether or not to cross it. I started out across it, and the neighbor said, "Yes, you can cross it." I got out about the middle of the creek, and the back end of the truck floated upward, and we just sat there while the wheels were spinning. Finally, my wheels "caught hold" on the rocks and out we came.

Alma New, Monticello, November 7, 2008

DETERMINED TEACHER

I remember the time some of the boys at school cut down a tree and it fell across the road on my route there. They did this so that I wouldn't come to school and they could be off that day.

I drove around the edge of the tree and got stuck in the mud. I walked to school and a neighbor got me out. One of my eighth-grade boys was furious with me for coming on to school. He thought for sure he was going to have a day off. He called the teacher's name that taught there the year before this. He said, "She would have just turned around and gone back home."

He also said that about the snow. If they happened to get caught there when it snowed, the teacher would turn them out and let them go home. But not me, as I stayed there for the rest of the day.

Joyce Campbell Buchanan, Barbourville, November 21, 2008

BRIDGE OUT AHEAD

In the summer of 1961 there had been a flood that washed out the walk bridge to the Pigeon School. For a bridge there remained a log with a few boards on top between two trees. We could walk over to the school rather easily until the debris fell into the creek below. By early October frost was making it [too] slick to walk without falling.

I went to the county superintendent's office and reported our bridge was almost impassable. They told me to go to the county judge to get a new bridge built. Nothing happened, so I went back to the school superintendent's office and informed them that I feared my one first grader, who was a six-year-old boy, would fall into the creek and perhaps drown before I got there in the mornings.

Nothing happened until November when the temperature dropped to twenty-two degrees and a light snow fell. I parked my car about one mile on the side of the blacktopped road and loaded my attendance book, lunch bag, the missionaries' Bible storybook, graded test papers, shoulder purse, and my long black coat on myself and walked on to the schoolhouse.

My first grader was safely inside the school with his big brother. They were there first because I had hired his big brother to build a fire in the potbelly stove each morning. I got halfway across the makeshift bridge and the next thing I know I'm underwater.

The children began crying and two older boys got in the creek and pulled me out some distance down the way. I had gone completely under the water, and even though I had learned to swim while going to Berea College, I had so many clothes on and they were so heavy I almost drowned. I walked back to my car, put my wet coat in the floor and drove to the superintendent's office, got out of my car, and the water poured on the street.

I walked upstairs and said, "Here's the first grader I feared might drown falling from that log at Pigeon School. Thank God it was me! I won't be back at Pigeon to teach until there is a new walk bridge, and I am going to insist I get paid for this day."

My watch went to the jeweler for drying and cleaning, and my wool coat went to the dry cleaners. That very afternoon, the school maintenance crew built a new bridge.

This story circulated all over our county. In a humorous vein, one of the comments was "Don't you know you are supposed to wait until summer to go swimming?"

Garnet Gay Bailey Goble, Flat Gap, January 20, 2009

WARM BUGGY

One weekend it was bitter cold when I was teaching in Caldwell County. I had gone home for the weekend, and when it was time for me to return it was snowing, and was also extremely cold. A father met me at the highway to take me in a buggy to the home where I was staying. He told me he had a surprise for me. He had heated some rocks and put them in burlap bags in the bottom of the buggy, and my feet stayed toasty warm.

Another time, at the same place I boarded, the water got up and the man brought his horse and wagon and took me out to the highway. The water was so high it slushed up into the wagon.

Loella Lowery, as told to Jeannine Moore, Dawson Springs,
January 10, 2009

Long Commute

One of the first boys I remember at Hamilton School was Terrell McPherson. He was in the first grade. His dad would ride him up partway to the school to meet me at the Hershel Hope family home, then we would walk from there together up the creek to the schoolhouse.

I lived with my parents here between Cyclone and Rock Bridge, and I rode a mule four or five miles to the Hamilton School, then kept the mule in Hershel Hope's barn all during the day. From there I'd walk with Terrell and some other kids up the branch to the school. All together, it took me about an hour to get to the school from where I lived.

Well, today Terrell McPherson is one of Monroe County's outstanding farmers. He lives in the Sulphur Lick community, and he and his son operate a dairy and probably milk four or five hundred cows. They have a very big operation.

J. Robert Miller, Rock Bridge, September 18, 2008

Horse and Car Collision

I had a good relationship with the kids. When I was driving to school, if I passed them I stopped to pick them up and let them ride. My daddy would worry about me, thinking I would get somebody hurt, get sued, and all that.

The bottom of my car was just ruined with mud from their shoes, but I just didn't have the heart to pass those kids up.

One afternoon we were driving out the road home and a horse was loose in the neighborhood and was there on the road. I thought he was far enough to my left that I could get around him. What happened is that one of my boys put his arm out the car window and hit the side of the car. That horse jumped against the car and made a big dent on my door on the driver's side.

That was one of my seventh-grade boys, but he also helped me change flat tires. I can't talk about him much!

Joyce Campbell Buchanan, Barbourville, November 21, 2008

Over the River and through the Woods

After teaching at Steep Hollow, I taught for one year at Temple Hill near Mammoth Cave National Park. In getting to this school I rode horseback, but the next year I had a car!

I had to ride that horse five or six miles each way to and from school. I always made it on time, thus was there at 8:00. I had to stay until 4:00 that afternoon, but I had to go through triple woods to get home, and it was almost dark when I'd go through there. I'd make Ole Dave speed up and really go fast through those woods! I mean, he was trotting fast.

I had to ride on Houchens Ferry to get across the river.

Blanche Demunbrun, Glasgow, September 30, 2008

Knee-Deep in Mud

During my third, fourth, and fifth years of teaching one-room schools in Carter County, I taught at a one-room school called Davy's Run. The school was located about two miles off Kentucky Route #1, near Hitchins, Kentucky. It was a good community, and I liked it very much. The people in the community were cooperative, and it seemed as if everyone thrived in harmony. However, there was one drawback! The dirt road was a mud hole during the winter and spring months. After rains, and especially after a thaw, the mud was literally knee-deep.

Most families owned jeeps. My husband worked it into his schedule to drive me to school in a three-quarter-ton truck, then come back to pick me up at the end of the day. I drove the dirt road myself without consequences on fair weather days.

Patricia Gibson, Greenup, April 11, 2009

Riding to Work

My first teaching job was at Oak Hill School where I had fifty-sixty students. They were all country kids, and they brought their lunches to school. I was living at home with my parents here in Rock Bridge at that time, so I rode a horse to school about four or five miles away.

I went up Skaggs Creek and came out at Persimmon, then went on to Oak Hill and put my horse in Hoover Wilson's barn during the day. Hoover would feed my horse at lunchtime.

If I were in a hurry to get to school, I'd let the horse trot. Well, something happened to my horse that year. My dad said I killed that horse riding it to school. That horse died after that.

During the winter when the weather was bad, I'd drive my father's car or truck.

Most all the kids walked to school back then. They carried their lunch buckets with them.

J. Robert Miller, Rock Bridge, September 18, 2008

Complicated Arrangements

To get to Union Hill School, you had to travel on a road that wound around and went up into the hills. But for me to get there as a teacher, I would drive to Victor Grider's house and park in their yard, then walk up the hill, climb over a fence, and go through the woods on this ridge in order to end up at school.

The Joe Jackson children, who were tenants on our farm, went to school where I was teaching. Sometimes I would meet them on my way to school in the morning, because they had a long walk. We'd walk together on to school.

When I taught at Bowman School, I drove my daddy's pickup truck, but I never did get stuck in a mud hole. I also walked a lot, too. If my dad needed his truck, he'd take me part of the way to school and let me out on top of Skaggs Creek hill, then I'd walk the rest of the way to school. That afternoon I'd walk back to the top of the hill at Skaggs Creek, and he'd meet me and take me on home.

When I drove Dad's pickup truck along the way I'd pick up other students—the Emberton kids, and a little Bowman girl, when they'd see me coming. If my truck hadn't passed their house, they knew I was going to walk, so here they'd come out and we'd walk along together. That afternoon after school we'd walk back together.

Betty Jane (Miller) Pence, Franklin, Tenn., September 29, 2008

Car Flipped Upside Down

One day, very early in the year, the county had just graded the road lead-ing to the school. It had rained hard the night before and on my way to school the next morning, I went over an embankment and flipped my car upside down. Although the two children in the car with me walked away without a scratch, I still bear the scar of thirteen stitches that I received for the gash in my leg.

After that, I got a horse named "Old Nell" and rode her until spring when the road was safer. Edwin A. Nethery lived near the school and he took care of my horse when I arrived in the morning. I will always remember how good he was to me and how much he helped to make my first year a success.

Hilda Snider, "Hilda Snider Recalls Teaching at Mitchell Run,"
Reflections, *February 2006*

Equine Experiences

I was going to ride this girl's horse since she wanted me to ride with her. So we lingered behind while the other students went on. After the others moved on she got her horse and saddle, and we got on it.

I got on the horse behind her, and it bucked us off!

I also rode a horse to high school, and when I got there I left my horse and saddle at the livery stable. We rented a stable near the school and put our horse up to be fed just so many ears of corn, but we'd feed the horse a bunch of corn!

Back then a lot of high school kids rode horses to school. Any of them that didn't live in Caneyville had to ride a horse to school, and that included most of them. When riding a horse down a muddy road, some-times the horse would slip and fall down. I've had all kinds of experiences.

I even rode a horse after I began teaching at a school in Butler County. Some of the time that I taught there I lived in Caneyville; sometimes I lived in Butler County. Or sometimes my parents took me to my grandparents' house over there, and I'd stay there while teaching during the week. I boarded there with them. They lived close enough to the school for me to walk, probably just one quarter of a mile. But when I'd want to come home on weekends, I rode my horse or one of theirs back home.

Bernice Shartzer, Caneyville, October 1, 2008

Big Fat Mule to the Rescue

This is a story about the time I was crossing Sinking Creek. Mr. Willie Turpin lived just on the other side of this great big creek, and every time it came a big rain that creek got so high I couldn't cross it with my horse. He had a big fat mule, and he said to me, "Now, when you can't cross the creek, just have your daddy bring you down to the creek, honk the horn, and I'll come over and get you."

Sure enough, the first big rain that came, my daddy took me down to the creek and honked his horn. Mr. Turpin came over on that big fat mule. I crawled up on the mule behind him and he took me on across, then I walked from there on down to the school. That was the biggest mule I ever saw!

Imogene Dick, Monticello, November 7, 2008

Grandpa Helps Out

The most secluded school at which I ever taught was at Norfork in Trimble County. All kids had to walk to and from school, and that was also true in all rural schools at which I taught. I picked up the ones that were on the road as I went to Nabb, Caldwell County. I drove from Farmersville on one side of Princeton, through Princeton, then on out to Nabb, a distance of about seventeen miles.

As I got closer to the school the students met me at the road and rode on to school with me.

Some of the kids walked all the way from home, and I guess it was a difficult situation during rainy times and cold weather. When I was going to a one-room school, I walked a mile to get there. When it was snowy or the weather was too bad, my grandfather would take us in a buggy or on horseback. If it were just pouring rain he took us to school in a buggy. He was a fine grandpa. His name was Billy McEntire.

Virginia DeBoe, Eddyville, October 7, 2008

Dressed Up and Ready to Ride

This is a story about how I got to school my first year, and that was at Cedar Hill. The school was about five miles from Big Sinking, where I lived. At that time I didn't have a car, and I didn't drive. The distance was too far to walk. Daddy bought me a big white horse that had big brown spots. It was a beautiful horse and we named it Ole Bob. He also bought me a saddle and some saddlebags.

I rode my horse to school that first day and left it at a neighbor's barn. He was Jack Denney. I had already talked with him about leaving my horse there, and he told me I was quite welcome to do it.

That morning I put my riding pants on, packed my dress and school supplies in my saddlebag, and took off to school. When I got down to Mr. Denney's barn he was waiting for me. He took my horse, unsaddled it, put the horse in a stable, then pitched some hay in there for my horse to eat that day.

I walked back up the hill to the Denney house, and Mrs. Denney was so very nice. She wanted me to change clothes in her parlor. I said, "No, I can do it at the barn."

She said, "No, you come on up here. There's nobody in that room, and I've never used it."

I took my saddlebag, went into her parlor, and changed from my riding pants to a pretty little school dress. I walked down the hill to school, which was just a short hop, skip, and jump over the hill to where the school was located.

When school was out that afternoon and I came back, Mr. Denney already had my horse saddled and ready for me to go. I stopped by Mrs. Denney's house and changed into my riding pants, packed my dress back in the saddlebag, then went down and got on my horse and rode back home.

Imogene Dick, Monticello, November 7, 2008

Wrong Side of the River

Each year I taught a one-room school at Elifha Creek, Camp Creek, and Allens Creek, I lived with a family on the wrong side of the river! I had to cross the river, and within the first six weeks I got a horse and rode it back and forth to school. That meant I had to also learn how to shoe my own horse and keep the horse clean. The kids loved my horse, and it was a spoken peace [proven] way to get in with the kids. It was also good because I went with the kids up the river to the school.

The kids would rub my horse down, and their fathers built a little shelter for my horse there at the three schools at which I taught. We moved to Stinking Creek, Knox County, where I partnered up with a nurse midwife from the Frontier Nursing Service. We started our own program on Stinking Creek in which she was going to deliver babies, and I was going to teach school so as to earn the money needed to support us.

I was viewed as a foreigner by Knox Countians when I moved to Stinking Creek. For punishment, or anything else, you were assigned to teach school located in a secluded location. That means it was a school that you couldn't get to in the wintertime. But that was alright with me because that was where I wanted to be in the first place.

In order to get to Stinking Creek in 1958, you had to step into the creek, walk in the water and out of the water at least ten to fifteen times in just one mile. I did have a horse, however, and most of the time I was able to ride it all the way to school. Sometimes I had to walk the whole distance.

Irma Gall, Barbourville, November 20, 2008

Hurt Feet

We had these roads that the WPA [Work Projects Administration] built and cared for by bedding them with big rocks that they beat into the ground. That was always a problem when I was going to school. In the summer we'd stump our toenails off and cry, and go on. And we'd also have those big stone bruises on our heels, and those bruises hurt just as bad as anything. They were just big blue blisters.

When it rained or snowed we'd sweep the schoolhouse to clean up the mud or snow. I've seen little kids that had to wait at a bus stop, but they had to walk a mile or more in order to get to the bus. They would be wringing wet. Sometimes, if they were fortunate enough, they would have an old pair of shoes to wear to the bus stop, and then put the clean pair on. However, many of those kids would come into school wet. When they took off their wet shoes, you could smell their feet.

Pat McDonald, Barbourville, November 21, 2008

Heading for Disappointment

When I was teaching at Disappointment, a one-room school which was locally called Pintment, in the wintertime you could not drive your car up every day, so I had to leave my car on Highway 11 at a friend's house and walk across a swinging bridge. The distance up to the schoolhouse was about one-half mile.

I have no idea why the school was named Disappointment.

Laura Agnes Townsley Stacy, Barbourville, November 21, 2008

Fallen First Grader

I recall walking a mile and one-half to get to Alex Creek School, and we crossed the creek thirteen times. The road was in and out of the creek. So this family at the mouth of the creek walked with me. We waded across the water and sometimes through the winter. I dropped the little first grader into the creek a few times. I had him on my back and was toting him across the creek and got him wet. I remember taking him inside the school and drying him up. We didn't turn around and go back home; we just went on to school.

I had enough money just to buy a pair of boots and a raincoat, so I wore those boots in the winter, and that's how I got across the creek.

Bige R. Warren, Barbourville, November 20, 2008

Fording the Creek

One of the little boys that was my brother's buddy lived on the bank of a creek, and when it rained and the creek got up, this little boy's mother would get us across the creek on a mule. She would take the mule down to the creek and hauled all of them across on the mule, but just one student at a time.

At that same school in February when the snow had begun to melt, we got down to the creek where you couldn't get across. Then I'd wade across, but first pulled my shoes off, then carried those two boys across the creek one at a time, and then put my shoes on the other side. My feet got so cold, it's a wonder I hadn't died, but it didn't kill me.

Joyce Williams Ward, Campbellsville, December 11, 2008

Bad Weather for Riding

On a cold, muddy day I rode my horse to school. Upon arrival, some boys put the horse in a nearby barn. By the end of the day clumps of mud and snow had frozen to the horse's feet. Wow, it was cold!

I was afraid to ride him home because I was scared that he might fall. Believe it or not, I led that horse for three miles to my parents' house.

Martha Campbell, Central City, December 13, 2008

LONG TRIP

My school day at Fairview began early for me, with a brisk walk across town from my mother's home to the intersection of Main Street and Bloomfield Road, where I would catch the outbound school bus. Mr. Summers, who was the regular driver, picked me up at 6:00 a.m. He would then go about ten miles out the Bloomfield Road and turn on a dusty, crushed stone road to Ashes Creek.

I rode with him for another five miles to a side "road" that was near my school. He would then continue on and make a loop through that part of the county, picking up ninth- through twelfth-grade kids to take to the town high school.

The county's one- and two-room schools accommodated first-through eighth-grade students. In the evening the driver would reverse his loop and pick me up on his way home after he had delivered the high school kids. We would return to town near suppertime.

The side "road" to Fairview School basically was a deeply rutted path that was passable only by vehicles with high road clearance. It ran about a half mile up the hill to the ridge where the school was located. The building and land belonged to a farmer who lived nearby.

Years later, when the school system was restructured, the school building became a barn. It was saddening to see its deteriorated condition when I took my teenage kids to see where their dad had taught "back in the dark ages."

William H. Nicholls Jr., The Villages, Fla., December 14, 2008

STORMY WEATHER

One day when going to school we had an awful storm and all the creeks were up. The mail carrier was still carrying a bell on a mule. When this man came to the school he said to me, "Are you afraid to ride behind me on this mule across the country?"

Well, this was different country so I said, "No, I'm not." So I got on that mule behind him and went across. When we got across there, some people were real busy and they had three big tubs full of cucumbers. They were canning those cucumbers. They said, "I think your schoolchildren aren't here yet."

This fellow said, "This weather here is awful stormy. It's too dangerous this stormy day." I rode back across the creek in a two-horse wagon, sitting on chairs. That was the longest trip in the world. My, what an experience! Thank God there are no more days like that.

Helen Raby, Elizabethtown, January 10, 2009

Chapter 9

Teacher and Community Relations

Most of the teachers who kindly contributed the stories for this book emphasize the central role played by the one-room school in the community. In these rural areas teachers routinely knew their students' parents, and often their extended families. It was not uncommon for teachers to be invited to students' homes for meals or even to spend the night.

A popular event in these communities was the annual pie supper, held to raise money for school supplies—but obviously attended sheerly for pleasure. Christmas programs were also common, and parents often attended ball games and other school events.

Among the stories below are a few that feature disgruntled parents, but they are the exception that proves the rule.

Community Events at the School

Pie suppers were popular, as were fiddlers' contests. For pie suppers, girls in the community would bring a homemade pie in a decorated box. The trustee, or some other man, would serve as auctioneer and raffle off the pies to the highest bidder.

Lots of teasing followed the bidding, but the money was used to purchase playground equipment, water buckets, ropes, and waste buckets. Sometimes a portable gas lamp, a globe, or a dictionary would be bought.

The whole community came for pie suppers, community plays, the Christmas program, and the Christmas tree. Everyone was interested in the teacher's gifts to each child.

Some parents came to watch the kids play in ballgames on Friday afternoon, and it was especially interesting to see that some parents came to get their children if a storm cloud appeared.

Mattie Jo Smith, Benton, March 7, 2009

Fund-raising and Beauty Contestant Pie Supper

The year I was at Oak Hill School we had a pie supper in order to raise some money to buy some equipment. We bought a volleyball net, and a volleyball, along with some recreational equipment. The school building was up on a hill, and this Ferguson boy hit that volleyball with his fist and knocked it all the way into the hollow.

Someone had to go get the volleyball. I criticized that Ferguson boy quite often for doing that. He is deceased now, as are a lot of other kids that went to school back then. However, they were all good country kids.

I still remember that annual pie supper. We had a big crowd; had some music, and an auction. The girls brought pies and the boys brought pocketbooks. We had a big time. I don't recall how much money we raised, but it was perhaps fifty to seventy-five dollars.

The auctioneer was Jack Wade, and he couldn't hear very well. He did a good job, though.

On occasion, two different boys wanted to buy the same pie since it was brought to be sold by a girl on whom both boys had a crush. So the pie supper was competitive, as the boys would compete with each other when buying their pies by bidding higher.

One thing I remember the kids competed in was a beauty contest. There was a girl who was put up in the beauty contest. My cousin William Denton Miller was there and he was backing this first girl. Then another girl was put up, and she was Dennis Page's girlfriend. Well, Dennis spent a lot of money on her.

I think that beauty contest was the most competitive thing we had. The boys had to pay a penny each time they voted. That wasn't much money for each vote, but money was scarce in those days.

We'd stand the girls up front to let the people look at them as they voted on them. People in the audience would cast their votes on the girl they wanted to be elected as the winner. The girls were usually pleased with what took place, as there weren't any hard feelings involved. It was a lot of fun, and it just cost one penny for each vote!

J. Robert Miller, Rock Bridge, September 18, 2008

Pie Suppers

We had pie suppers at school as a way to make money needed to buy crayons and different things for the school, such as construction paper, balls and bats for the kids to play with. We had to have ways of making some money for the schools, because we didn't get money from the board of education for things like that.

We raised the pie supper money in different ways. For example, the girls would bring in decorated boxes with food in them, sometimes pies, and the boxes would be auctioned off. Boyfriends especially bid on them as they were being auctioned off by someone in the community. The girls names were not on the boxes, but the boys would always find out who brought them. Then when they'd sell each box, they'd set it down and put the girl's name on it, and who bought it.

When I went to school, we also had pie suppers. Funny things happened at pie suppers. My sister's box got stolen one time at Mosby's Ridge, where she went to school. Anyway, because the boy that wanted it didn't get it, he had somebody to steal it and run off with it, but they finally found it several days later!

We took boxes up there to that school to help them out. Those boxes were auctioned off at different amounts, but sometimes they'd be sold for as much as five dollars. That was really something. My daddy's cousin Ralph Estes was always going to pie suppers and auctioning boxes off. He was good. He also auctioned at house sales, and at other things.

Virginia Janes, Edmonton, September 22, 2008

IMPORTANCE OF PIE SUPPERS AT SCHOOL

At these pie suppers, the girls would bring the pie, but their names were not placed on the bottom of the box. Information as to who put a pie or candy in the box was passed around secretly. They used numbers instead of names as a means of identifying whose box it was.

I remember at our pie supper at Union Hill, I was dating this boy, and he came. Somebody else knew when my pie was being auctioned off, so they started running the price up on him and he ended up having to pay about six dollars. That was a lot of money then! That was always the joke to find out which pie was the teacher's.

If a pie brought one or two dollars, that was standard. All total, there were usually twenty or twenty-five pies there.

For that night, my dad built a stand outside with four boards around a square. We'd have candy bars, ice cream, and chewing gum to sell. A cone of ice cream was sold for a nickel. We had strawberry, vanilla, and chocolate ice cream, but my dad had to go buy it; thus we had to pay for the ice cream. That was a big treat for children out in the country to get to buy ice cream.

If you made thirty dollars that night, it brought in a lot of money for the school to spend for needed things.

Betty Jane (Miller) Pence, Franklin, Tenn., September 29, 2008

Cotton Pie

We had a pie supper at the Mattingly School where I taught, and it was just more than I wanted to undertake, both before and after it took place. As to what took place at a pie supper, young ladies in the community made pies, and most of them had boyfriends, and the boys had to bid on their girlfriend's pie until he got it. The pies were auctioned off by a local auctioneer.

One girl made a pie and put a female friend's name on it. It was a cotton pie! It had only cotton in it. Well, the boy bought it, and he had a cotton pie. That girl made that pie as a joke. It may have been that she was jealous of the girl whose name she put on the pie. [*Laughter*]

I just had the one pie supper, but had a big crowd, and most of the girls made pies. But that pie supper was just too confusing to suit me.

Mayola Graves, Loretto, September 9, 2008

Pie Suppers at Steep Hollow School

I remember when we had pie suppers. My dad would let me take a pie, but he'd never let me compete for the most important player [contest] for girls that night—the best-looking girl. He never would let me run for that.

If you ran for that, they'd give you so much money that counted for your beauty points as to whether you'd win or not. He never would let me do that.

See, whichever boy that bought your pie had to take you home. He'd [my dad] always manage for someone else to buy my pie.

The boys knew whose pie it was, because the auctioneer always told whose it was. Sometimes there would be two or three boys that bid on a pie. Sometimes a pie might sell for five dollars, and that was a lot of money back then. The auctioneer told whose pie it was, hoping that two or three bidders would compete with each other.

The school used the pie supper money . . . to buy things like notebooks, tablets, pencils, crayons, and other types of materials that would be used there in school.

Blanche Demunbrun, Glasgow, September 30, 2008

Stolen Watermelon

Every school had to do something that would raise money for the school. The thing we had was an ice cream supper. My mama and daddy helped me get all the ice cream together, and one of their friends helped them.

We all went to the school that night, and while I was taking care of other things in the building and outside, the school had an ugly man contest, pretty girl contest, guess the identity of the pie, sold tickets on a watermelon, and all kinds of things like that. I was back and forth taking care of things like that. Mama and Daddy sold the ice cream they had purchased while all that was taking place. They bought it to help the school, because they both worked every day and could afford to do it.

We had this great big watermelon setting outside the door on a table where everybody could see it, and I was selling tickets on it. Then we drew names to see who won the watermelon. By golly, when we went out to get the watermelon, it was gone!

[*Laughter*] We didn't know who took it, but somebody stole it, and the one that drew the name as the winner, I had to pay them.

Years later I heard that it was Woodrow Wilson that took the watermelon, and I didn't doubt it a bit! [*Laughter*]

I think the watermelon tickets cost a dollar, but it might have been fifty cents. Whatever it was, the same amount was charged persons who guessed what kind of pie for which they were buying tickets.

We took the money that we got that night. I think it was about seventy dollars, and I was real proud of it. We used that money to get the building painted. We were hoping to make enough to drill a well, but we didn't make enough money for that.

Billie Sue Blakeman, Edmonton, September 22, 2008

The Romance of the Pie

For pie suppers, mothers would bake pies and bring them. A parent in that family, usually the father, would hold the pie up for everyone to see, then auction it off. They took bids on it, and the person that bid the highest got the pie.

It often happened that two boys bid on the pie in competition with each other, because they both liked the girl!

I met my husband at a pie supper at Coles Bend. I wasn't teaching there then, but he had dated the teacher who was there. He came to see her, but pretty soon she introduced him to me! After that we started courting each other. He kissed me pretty soon after that!

Our grandkids get a kick out of that story.

Virginia Galloway, Merry Oaks, December 3, 2008

Illegal Ice Cream

We decided that a traditional ice cream supper was to be held to raise some funds for the school. I had never been connected with an ice cream supper and did not know the county health department requirements for such an event. During the early planning stages for the event it seems as though I was overlooking the small fact that we did not have the requisite running water at the school. Fortunately for me the problem surfaced early enough to be avoided, thanks to my grandfather, an attorney in town, who knew the regulations and smoothed things out with the health department before it became a reportable offense.

After discussing the issue with him, we decided not to have a fund-raiser. Instead we had a very successful "meet and greet," sans ice cream. That way we could skirt their rules completely. Many of the parents who attended brought picnic-style home cooking and desserts that were out of this world. Thanks, Pop.

William H. Nicholls Jr., The Villages, Fla., December 14, 2008

Annual Christmas Programs

We had a Christmas program every year. One year when we were having the program, there were two religious factions from the same church that were there because their kids were there. One faction always knelt down when they prayed, but the others didn't.

When we had our Christmas program and got ready to pray, I said, "Let's stand to pray." But I didn't know there were two factions in the church. Well, the faction that didn't believe in standing to pray, but believed in kneeling to pray, was not happy.

The Christmas program didn't take place in that church, it's just that the church was predominant in that community. However, the church's members were of two different minds.

Bernice Shartzer, Caneyville, October 1, 2008

Christmas at School

They always had a Christmas program at this rural school. The children would recite Christmas verses. Their parents were always there, and their presence made a packed house.

We didn't have electric lights back then. We had little candles that they would clip on the trees, and we had trees that caught on fire lots of times! We'd put them out real fast.

I remember this story when I was going to school to my uncle Russell, who was the teacher. He'd put candles all over the tree, and we'd spend our time trying to put out the fire from the candles.

When we'd have these Christmas programs, we'd sing Christmas carols, and the parents would come every year to see all of that. The parents were pretty easy to get along with. I never did have any bouts with any of the parents in the rural schools.

Virginia Janes, Edmonton, September 22, 2008

Outstanding Lifetime Memory

These children [at Denney Hollow] loved any dramatic work and really wanted to prepare a large Christmas program for the parents. We worked for weeks learning songs, poems, and a large play. The date for the program was set, and the previous day was a day that looked as though we might not have school or program or anything the next day.

That night it snowed about six to eight inches. I didn't know if anybody could get there, but I went on and built a fire in the stove and got the place warm. Immediately people came walking or in wagons, sleds, and pickup trucks until the room was filled. The children performed beautifully, and to this day when I meet one of them they mention that Christmas program.

That event was an outstanding memory of a lifetime!

Lucille Hoover Ringley, Monticello, March 24, 2009

TRADING GIFTS FOR CHRISTMAS

For Christmas gift time, we always had a cedar tree in the corner of our classroom. The children decorated it with construction-paper chains made by gluing strips together. When it came time to do it, they drew names to exchange gifts, but not everyone was happy with the name they drew. Sometimes trading names took place.

They brought their gifts the day we dismissed for Christmas holiday, and the teacher brought them a treat bag, including an apple, orange, banana, stick candy, and gum. For those children out in the country, that was a special treat! Can you imagine children today being excited when they get that?

Betty Jane (Miller) Pence, Franklin, Tenn., September 29, 2008

SANTA CLAUS

My sister, Betty Jane, taught at Bowman School, located close to here. I was in college at that time. She was living at home with our parents, and I lived here in this house. When it came Christmas time, she asked me to be her Santa Claus. Well, I dressed up like Santa and got up in the back of a pickup truck. Betty Jane had all the goodies there that we called "treat."

They were having a Christmas party at the Bowman School; had a Christmas tree and were going to give out "treat" and have Santa Claus there. So I got in the back of the pickup truck and rode down through the Rock Bridge community. While passing through I waved at everybody. I was wearing white gloves, had on a Santa Claus face, a red suit, and I scared the dickens out of everybody. They'd yell, "Oh, there goes Santa Claus!"

I went on over to the Bowman School, and had the time of my life. They had a lot of fun as I passed out gifts to the students. I really had a ball!

J. Robert Miller, Rock Bridge, September 18, 2008

SINKS FOR CHRISTMAS

One of the things that really got the attention of parents right away is that at Christmas time we had nothing but a water bucket and a dipper, and also a little table for the family. With the help of a friend, I was able to get hold of a bunch of old cast-iron sinks they were throwing away up in the Bluegrass area.

My friend would go collect them, and I'd take one to school. We'd make a little table and put that sink in there, then put a drain down, and the water disappeared! We didn't have to open a window and throw it out. I would do this during the first month in school when I was teaching there. Then by the second week here comes a mother who wanted to see how that works. It was fabulous, because there was no mud puddle out there. She asked, "Where did the water go?"

I told her we dug a drain out toward the creek, or out in the road somewhere, and we'd dig a pit and fill it up with rocks before the kids could get all of that. Then I would go to the parents and tell them that for five dollars we would install a sink. I got the parents' attention on that.

Irma Gall, Barbourville, November 20, 2008

Special School Performances

We would take sheets and string wires across the stage. The sheets were put up for curtains so we could have plays on the stage. So many people would come to the schoolhouse that many of them had to stand up and lean against the walls while the play went on.

I don't recall why we did this, but we always sang wherever I taught. At Christmas time we'd always sing Christmas songs and put on a good program. We'd even dress up like different characters.

Literature was always dear to my heart, so these plays and songs went right along with my teaching.

Anna Smith Collins, Marion, November 20, 2008

Kickbacks

The students all walked to school. However, I began to stop on my way and ask families of students to ride with me. It was a dirt road and was traveled only by a very few automobiles. When it got colder, those farm families butchered a hog and I became a recipient of a large brown bag of pork tenderloin.

When I took it home my dad, a school supervisor for our county at that time, shook his head and said, "Oh no, honey. You can't start accepting bribes, or 'kickbacks.' That's against the law. You will have to return this."

I believe that was my first experience with the realization that one could be fired from his/her job for accepting a favor from a student's parent. However, I did not return the gift!

Garnet Gay Bailey Goble, Flat Gap, January 20, 2009

Just Talk

At Bee Spring, which was the first two-room school at which I taught, the teacher that taught with me was Nelda Wood. She just about knew everybody over there, and she helped me an awful lot.

One day some lady said, "The minute that she [Demunbrun] get here and gets my boy, I'm going to really get her."

Well, her son was the first one I had to discipline.

Nelda then said to me, "Well, she didn't come and get all over you." I said, "I never did see her." So, I guess that mother was just talking!

Blanche Demunbrun, Glasgow, September 30, 2008

Death Threat

I had one parent here in town that threatened to kill me, to cut my throat. That happened down at the old school building here, in which we had a week's duty for so many teachers from first grade through high school. Every time it was your time, you had early duty and had to be there by 6:00 in the morning. Your job was to take care of all the kids coming in from all the buses. And every afternoon you stayed there on duty until every bus ran. If the bus broke down, you stayed there with the students. And I had their names written down, which bus they were to get on, and every afternoon when it was time to go to the bus, I'd line them all up to get in line for the bus.

Well, it was late that afternoon, and I was sitting there waiting to get to go home. A car drove up, and this man and woman asked, "Where's my boy?" I said, "Well, I put him in line with his bus."

"Well, he didn't get off the bus. He's not there at home. I'm going back home, and if he's not there, I'm going to come back and cut your throat. I'm going to kill you, and I'm going to kill Thomas Butler [the superintendent]."

I was scared to death. I didn't know what in the world to do. I called Thomas Butler at home and told him what was happening. He said, "Stay down there and wait. Maybe the boy got on the wrong bus. Maybe they'll bring him back."

I walked up to town, which wasn't far from the school. My daddy sold insurance, and I told him, "I'm scared to death. He threatened to kill me." Then I told him who it was.

He said, "You go back down there and stay. I'll see about this."

I went back down there, and my little cousin went with me. We sat in the car and waited and waited; then I thought, "Oh, my Lord, what am I going to do?"

After awhile Daddy drove up and said, "It's alright now. You can go home."

I said, "Daddy, what happened?"

He said, "That little boy saw his two half sisters." They were half sisters who were in high school. The little boy saw them lined up to get on the bus, and then he went over and got on the bus and went home with them.

The boy's mother had left her husband and all the children and went to live with another man, and then they had this little boy. Well, when he saw his half sisters, he just went and got in their bus line and they let him go home with them.

Daddy knew the people, so he went to the home that the boy was supposed to have gone to. Then he went to the other house, and the little boy was there with his half sisters instead of where he was supposed to be. They went and got him.

I was scared to death during all of that, because this man was so mean. He was from a very, very mean family.

As a coincidence, I went to Dollar General Market and looked at this man standing there with white hair and mustache. When I saw him I said, "You look familiar."

He kind of grinned. I called his name, and that was the boy that went with his two stepsisters that day.

That really happened.

Billie Sue Blakeman, Edmonton, September 22, 2008

WRONGLY ACCUSED

I only remember one occasion when I was criticized. After teaching a lesson on personal hygiene, there was a parent that wrote a letter to the Pike County Board of Education complaining that I was trying to tell the children how and when to take a bath, how to brush their teeth, and what kind of clothes to wear.

A supervisor mentioned the letter to me, but only in a very professional way, and assured me to worry nothing about the complaint and to continue with the good job I was doing at the rural school. The letter of complaint had been exaggerated, because I had never told the children what kind of clothes to wear.

Stella K. Marcum, Pikeville, February 10, 2009

Bad Neighbor

I didn't have to spank children at Penick School very much. They were pretty good. Their families were religious. One of the things I recall that took place was that we played pretty rough outside, and a neighbor lived up on the hill. She didn't like it because I was teaching there, due to the fact her friend used to teach there but didn't want to anymore.

This lady told a big tale claiming the kids had tied me to a tree. Some of the kids was laughing about it and said, "We didn't do that. Why did she tell that?"

She was kin to some of the kids, and I knew the lady. What it was all about is that she thought we were playing rough, but shouldn't have been.

Virginia Janes, Edmonton, September 22, 2008

Mom Helps Out

There was a mother of two kids that lived close to the school. She would always come and stay with the kids at school if I ever had to take a sick kid home. She'd look after one of the kids if he/she got sick while I was gone. Usually I'd just take a sick kid home, but on one occasion I did take one to a doctor.

That happened back when the school building had burned. Due to the fire, there was a piece of metal sticking out. The kids ran barefooted back then, and one of these children cut her foot really bad—cut a big spot in her toe and it was bleeding really badly.

I had to take her to a doctor because I couldn't get hold of her parents. I brought her into town to a doctor, and my friend across the street, Mary Carter, stayed with other students until I returned.

Zona Royse, Columbia, October 4, 2008

MISSIONARY VISITATIONS

Each Thursday afternoon the Assembly of God missionaries would visit the school to lead the students in songs and finger plays. They would tell and illustrate a Bible story on a flannel board. They had excellent skills in illustration.

We were given a Bible verse to memorize for the next week. All the students took this seriously. It was a great asset, a break from monotony, and a positive emotional outlet to the isolation in our mountain communities.

Betty Jo Arnett Lykins, Salyersville, February 9, 2009

IMPRESSIVE FUNERAL SERVICE

The funeral director of a local funeral home contacted me one day at school and said, "Noble, I wish you would conduct a funeral service for an infant baby tomorrow up here at the church. The family is poor, and they are not going to be able to have a minister, so will you conduct that?"

I said, "Man, I never conducted one in my life, but I've been to many funerals and I have no idea how long I've been a pallbearer, but you asked me something I don't know about?"

He looked at me, and I had known him all my life, and he said, "You will do it, won't you?"

I said, "I'll try."

So this is what I thought about that afternoon and that night. The next morning, I'd gotten the students out there, and thank goodness it was a beautiful day. I lined them up in three rows and told them what we were going to do.

A lot of those seventh- and eighth-grade boys and girls were church members, and they sang at church every Sunday and in some prayer meetings. They could sing and could really harmonize it. So I designated one of them to be in charge of the program. I said, "You can lead the singing and you can have a scripture reading, then close with the Lord's Prayer and an appropriate song."

That just tickled the students to death, and we marched up there in a single file and went into the church. When we got inside, I said to the funeral director, "When you get up to turn over the church service, turn it over to this student, and she will be in charge."

The funeral director did his part, then said, "So-and-so is now in charge of the funeral service."

Now, you talk about something impressive—I shall never forget it, the students will never forget it, and the people there in attendance will never forget it. For years I'd meet up with someone I had in school or some of their parents, and they'd say, "Mr. Noble, you know, I never will forget that funeral program. It was so impressive."

I said, "Well, I give the credit to all the students because they did it all."

They'd say, "That's what made it impressive. The girl doing the leading was only in the eighth grade."

I said, "That's right."

Noble H. Midkiff, Whitesville, December 1, 2008

School Fair

There were not many students there at Nabb School, but it was a wonderful place to teach. With no more than fourteen students, we had time to do projects and different special things. One of the things we did, we had a school fair. We had science projects that taught them about seeds and distribution, and all those kinds of things.

We made posters and pottery, and some artwork like painting gourds and things like that. Doing all those things developed into a school fair to which they all brought their vegetables and other things like that, and they were judged. It was just a fun day.

Neighbors and patrons all gathered in.

Virginia DeBoe, Eddyville, October 7, 2008

Community Service

In those days Carter County schools had a "School Daddy" program. Davy's Run School had two older respectable businessmen who served in that capacity. They would oversee the building and goings-on at school. Occasionally they would visit school and observe classes. Sometimes they would speak to the group, and often bring the children a treat.

That program was accepted well during those years, and in my opinion it was a valuable asset to the one-room schools in Carter County.

We would hang sheets across an area of the room and present a Christmas play for the community. It was always well attended. Students would draw names from a box and give the recipient a gift. It was a fun place to be and a highlight in the community.

One beneficial and enjoyable part of the school was the "traveling library." A well-known schoolman in the administration was Mr. Ercel Kozee. He would bring the wooden chest filled with an assortment of books, and the day he arrived was like a holiday for many students. They were excited to get into the box and view the new books. After the books had been read and swapped around, we would notify Mr. Kozee and he would arrive with a new set of books. Needless to say, he was a welcome visitor.

At the end of each month, I would give prizes for attendance. Each student received something, and the perfect attendance students received something extra.

Miss Grace Pond, a missionary, would visit each month and illustrate a Bible story on the flannel board. This was acceptable in all county schools, and was enjoyed by students.

Patricia Gibson, Greenup, April 11, 2009

VISITING HOURS

On Friday afternoons at Bowman School, mothers, babies, and little brothers and sisters would come and sit in the classroom just to observe what we were doing. This wasn't every week, but that happened several times.

It was good that they were there, because it taught the little kids what their older brothers and sisters were doing there at school.

On Friday afternoons we used to have ciphering matches and spelling bees. And they really liked to come and watch these things.

Betty Jane (Miller) Pence, Franklin, Tenn., September 29, 2008

PARENTS WELCOME

Sometimes parents came to school to talk about situations that were maybe developing, but most often they came just to visit. They also came for programs being held at school. About three times a year they would bring picnic lunches and have a big feast at the noon hour. All of them just spread out what they brought so that all parents and kids could share with each other.

Their kids always looked forward to having their parents there, especially with the lunches. When that took place, it was always dignified and common manners displayed.

Anna Smith Collins, Marion, November 20, 2008

Lasting Relationships

As I was teaching my first year, the schoolroom needed painting. The county would furnish the paint after some arm-twisting. My husband did the repair, wash, painting, etc. But this one time he was so busy that I let three or four high school boys paint the room. They were older brothers of some of the students.

After the painting was over I furnished food for a picnic, using our classroom and our first grade table. Some of the parents were so pleased they came to the picnic.

These one-room schoolchildren remain very close to me, especially those in the first school at which I taught for eight years. Some of them still call to see how I'm doing since my husband died June 8, 2008.

One of my first graders, the one who climbed a tree and fell, lost his mother to cancer, called me to let me know he was coming back to Kentucky and wanted to see me. Sadly, he didn't get to come because his cancer was back. He and his brother and sister have cancer, and their mother and father both died from cancer.

These children from the one- and two-room schools are the ones who still keep in contact with me. Once a year at Fish Trap Lake we have a picnic called the One-Room School Picnic. We all, students and I and two friends, are there. An announcement was put in the local papers. This has been done for the last four or five years. The first picnic was attended by about three hundred, but not as many last year.

Pauline Keene Looney, Pikeville, December 8, 2008

Breakfast with Families

While I was teaching at Breezeel, many of the parents invited me to spend the night with the family. Fried potatoes, molasses, and homemade biscuits and gravy were on the breakfast menu.

One little third-grade girl whispered to me when she came up for class that she had made the biscuits for the family breakfast that morning.

Mattie Jo Smith, Benton, March 7, 2009

Sleepovers

Our teacher was in her twenties when she married, which was considered late. She lived a mile or two from the schoolhouse with her parents and younger sister. If we students were good all week, once in a while the teacher would let one of us go spend the night with her and her family.

I only did that once, but I don't know if this was because I was a relative, or just naughty at times. But I do know that Daddy said, "If you get a spanking at school, you just might get one when you get home."

Pauline Keene Looney, Pikeville, December 8, 2008

Benevolent Deed

One cold winter I was teaching at Sims Creek School in my home community. During those years you did not face the same fears we experience today. For instance, all the children walked safely to school without worry that someone would be hit by a car. One of the greatest blessings was never hearing about a child being sexually molested, or people using drugs.

An older couple from Virginia moved into our community. Each evening about dark we would see them walking by our home. We became quite curious, saying to each other, "Why do they go by at this time every day?" My mother asked our neighbors, who told her that the couple had to go to their niece's house at night because they needed food, a warm place to sleep, etc. My mother felt immediate compassion and said, "I will look for them tomorrow and I'll invite them to come and spend the night."

So that's what she did. They were really thrilled when Mother invited them, and gladly replied, "We will be there tomorrow evening." My parents, brothers, and I welcomed Mr. and Mrs. McVey upon arrival.

Later I said to Mother, "I want my students to do something especially nice for Mr. and Mrs. McVey." I knew that my students' parents were kind and always eager to lend a helping hand. The next day at school I announced to my thirty-five students that we had an elderly couple in need of food, then I asked, "Do any of you have an idea what we can do?"

One of my very thoughtful students spoke up, "Oh, I know what we can do!"

I replied, "Mary, tell us."

Mary said, "All of us can bring food from our homes."

I said, "Oh, that is a great idea! We all should practice benevolence. Let's make a list of various foods that we can bring from our homes to our schoolroom." We went on and made a list on the chalkboard, writing down such items as potatoes, onions, canned food, pinto beans, pickles, jam, canned apples, molasses, eggs, etc. Then Johnny said, "Mother will let me stop at Tulie Bishop's store and purchase something."

I went on with the plans by asking, "When can you bring your food?" Their reply was "Tomorrow." Then I asked the students how we would get the food to the McVeys' home after it was brought to school. A handsome eight-year-old boy piped up, "After we get our food here, we can invite them to school." I further explained to the students as how this was a great example of benevolence, because we all were showing compassion to someone in need. However, we agreed to keep our plans a secret until they arrived.

The next morning was an exciting time! All of my students walked three-fourths to one and one-half miles each way to school, and here they came with a smile on their face and a sparkle in their eyes as they handed me the food that they carried so carefully. Then I noticed that the two little girls that lived one and one-half miles away had not arrived yet. I began getting concerned, thinking that their mother must be very ill again and they would have to miss school today. Within a few minutes in walked Iris, age eight, and her little sister Bethanie, age six, with a very sad expression on their face. Iris looked at us with tears in her eyes and said, "I dropped my half gallon of green beans, and they broke." We did not criticize them; instead the other students reassured the girls that this was alright.

Now the food was all gathered but we needed to plan how and when to present it to Mr. and Mrs. McVey, the grandparents of two of our students, Ray and Clarice. Ray spoke up, "We can walk home with Grandfather and Grandmother and carry these products for them." All the students liked this idea. I asked the students to bring a note from their nice parents granting permission to carry their food to the McVeys' house, reminding them we would only walk to the boat landing and not actually get in the boat. Each parent sent me permission for their child to help with carrying the food.

That afternoon after I got home I began looking for the McVeys to go by at their usual time. I saw them coming so I went up to the gate and said, "My students and I want to invite you to our school at 2:00 p.m. on Friday. We will sing for you. We love to sing religious songs. You will also have an opportunity to meet your grandson's friends." Then I asked, "Will you come?" The answer was, "Thank you, Miss Thacker, for the invitation."

On Friday my students became very restless at 1:30 p.m. They couldn't wait to see Ray and Clarice's grandparents. They were so proud of their efforts to help someone less fortunate. Promptly at 2:00 I heard a knock. I walked to the front door and greeted the McVeys with a handshake to show them that they were really welcome. I said, "All of these boys and girls are happy to meet you." Then we sang several church songs that people in our community sung. Afterwards I asked, "Mr. McVey, will you lead us in prayer?" He gladly accepted and he, along with Mrs. McVey, began praying quite loudly while down on their knees. The children and I bowed our heads.

One of the things we did at school every morning was to recite the Lord's Prayer together as a group. So to my surprise Iris began trying to repeat every word that Mr. McVey was saying. She really thought she was supposed to. I'm sure that she had never been to a public church or worship service.

When the prayer was over I told the McVeys, "We have a great surprise for you. Look this way at the table." Their eyes expressed the surprise! They had no idea that we were going to give them much-needed food. They were overjoyed! I explained that all thirty-five of the students had contributed and that everyone was going to walk down the road with them, as far as the boat landing, to help carry their bounty.

The entire class began walking that mile down the road, laughing and talking, because we felt so thankful that we were doing a great benevolent act. The class said good-bye, leaving a very happy Mr. and Mrs. McVey on the riverbank to ride their boat across. We all walked back to school, where it was time to dismiss.

Several years have passed but I continue to treasure the memories of that happy event when my class and I were able to express benevolence to a needy couple.

Christine Thacker Justice, Mt. Sterling, February 18, 2009

Chapter 10

Students with Special Needs

In the era of the one-room schoolhouse there were no special education classes for children with special needs, nor was there any training for their teachers. As indicated by the stories that follow, however, teachers rose to the occasion as best they could; as one teacher put it, of primary importance was "care for people," a hallmark of the one-room school era.

Useful Contribution

When I taught at one school, I had a kid that was somewhat mentally disabled, and that was in the days of no special education. We kept finding crayons in a pencil sharpener every day, and he would volunteer to clean the pencil sharpener. So I discovered that he was the child that was putting the crayons in the pencil sharpener.

He really just couldn't do much of anything, although he was about sixteen and pretty well grown. But they had church in this little school building on Sunday, and the church people would sort of hide their wood so we wouldn't burn it. I guess I took a hatchet or something, but anyway I discovered that he knew how to use that. He would split the wood for us to make kindling to use in starting a fire. So, we got to leaving kindling beside the stove on Friday, along with maybe a wastebasket of paper for them to use in starting their fire on Sunday. They left us a new hatchet.

That gave this boy something to do, so the crayons stopped getting into the pencil sharpener after that!

I'd seen my mother deal with mentally disabled students. She'd say, "Well, if they have the gray matter between their ears, I can teach them, but if they don't, I can't."

Zona Royse, Columbia, October 4, 2008

STUTTERING CURE

One of my boys that was in the fifth grade where I taught in Crittenden County was Jimmy King, and he stuttered terribly. I told him one day, "Jimmy, would you mind giving up a little time of your recess and let me work with you?"

He said, "Yes, ma'am, I'll be glad to."

I said, "Jim, I don't know what it is. I don't know if it's a fear of your teacher or what, but I don't want you to be afraid of me. I do want you to respect me, but I want us to slow down and we're going to work on your stuttering to see if we can help you."

By the end of that year, that boy was not stuttering.

Emma Walker, Eddyville, October 7, 2008

UNABLE TO LEARN

When I taught at Red Cross, I had a little boy who just simply couldn't do schoolwork. He'd come to school, and part of the time he'd stay in a seat, but he would often get up and leave the room without permission and go outside.

I don't know how he knew when to go out, but the children would all get upset and tell me that he was out there on the slide.

We had some sleigh ride equipment that he was on, and those kids would say, "He's going to get hurt. He's going to get hurt."

What he did would upset the whole room of students. When he did that, I'd either go out to stop him or ask the principal to send somebody to get him.

He never learned to read or anything. He'd use a book, but he didn't know how to write on paper, so he'd just sit at his desk, tear up paper, and throw it on the floor.

I had a little girl student that didn't learn very well. She was more capable of being disciplined than the boy. She wouldn't study, but I'd give her a page to learn, and I'd tell her to work on certain words, then give her some directions as to what the words were.

If she couldn't do what I told her to do, she'd just tear the page out of the book. I remember spanking her a time or two for doing that.

There were others that had problems but those two were the most difficult that I remember. Of course, in those days we had no special aid classes.

Virginia Galloway, Merry Oaks, December 3, 2008

GIRL WITH DOWN SYNDROME

I had a Down syndrome child. At that time we did not have any special classes in our one-room schools for children with special needs. If they came to school, the only thing they had to do was just to come and be with the others.

Mildred had a good memory, and she could talk. She loved using spelling flash cards, and she could spell a lot of words. She learned math facts and how to solve math problems, and also learned a lot of other things.

One day the maintenance men were there working. They were painting the outside of the school building, and they had a bucket of paint setting out on the playground. We went out for recess, and she did something that I didn't know about at the time. She got into the paint bucket and she just stirred and stirred and stirred that paint, then she took the lid off of their water cooler and stirred up their water cooler with that paintbrush!

These men weren't too alarmed about what she did, and were very nice about it.

Imogene Dick, Monticello, November 7, 2008

BOY WITH DOWN SYNDROME

During my second year of teaching, this time at Valley Grove, I had a Down syndrome boy, who was nine or ten years old. We had no special education programs in the county at that time, so most such students did not attend school at all.

This boy came to school with an older sister and I think the process was very beneficial for him. I was not able to give him much individual attention. However, there were times when I tried to teach him how to print his name, and he would seem to be making progress. But the next day he would be back to square one.

He probably gained more from the contacts with other students than he did from me.

Grover C. Garland, London, December 26, 2008

SPECIAL PROBLEMS

I had a child with epilepsy. When she had a "spell," she just stiffened up and fell backward, chair and all. I'd make sure she had something between her teeth and see to it that she didn't swallow her tongue. We'd all be very concerned. She also had a learning problem.

Another child had a severe speech problem. When he read I could only judge by the inflection of his voice if he were reading correctly. Speech classes were not held, or help given in my college courses. This child was highly intelligent. He now has a doctorate degree in nuclear medicine. I spoke with him a year or so ago, and he mentioned, without a speech problem, that his son also had had speech problems, but had been in speech therapy and taken care of.

Betty Holmes McClendon, Nancy, January 26, 2009

UNDERSTANDING HUSBAND

My first experience with a mentally retarded student was during my first year in special education in Crittenden County. I had seven students, and I walked in there having never been around mentally retarded children. I had gone to school at Murray that summer, trying to get prepared as well as I could.

You talk about a shock to your system; that was a shock to me. But after I went into it, my motto was that "quitters never win." I said to myself that I had started something, and can't back down now.

My husband, Doyle, went with me my first semester at Murray College, and sat in on the special education classes just to see and to get an idea of what I was going to go through. He did get the idea as to what it would be like for me, and what I'd be facing during years to come. That way he could support me.

Miss Billie Downing was my teacher, and she will never forget it. She used Doyle as an example, I guess for as long as she taught at Murray, as to how he supported me. That was really going the extra mile.

Emma Walker, Eddyville, October 7, 2008

SPECIAL ED KID MAKES GOOD

When I moved to DeWitt Elementary School in 1967, the principal gave me what then were the first special education kids. I had fifteen or sixteen of those kids, and there was one kid who was in special education, but he was probably smarter than we'd all thought.

He was a kid that you just couldn't control. He would just take a notion to leave and go home any second. If recess was in session, you might miss him. The principal said to me, "I'm going to give him to you and I want you to take him and see what you can do with him."

The boy was actually a neighbor of mine. I took him and called him by name, then said, "If you will learn one word a day and do me one math problem a day, and learn to write your name, you'll pass my class, and you and I will be friends here."

When I got him, he quit that running away. But I watched him later, and that's why this story comes to mind. He didn't go but another year or two, then quit school. He got a job with a coal mining company later on, and one day I ran into him. He told me, said, "Bige, I just want to thank you for teaching me how to write my name. Now I can sign my own check."

I said, "Well, if you don't mind comparing your salary with my salary, let's do it."

As I had assumed, he made more money than I made!

He is still a good friend. He works on my automobiles occasionally now, and he can make a car. He can do anything to a car, and anything relative to coal mining. He could fix any machinery they have, so they paid him well. He worked for them for ten years or so. He is presently retired, and still does cars and a little mechanical work on the side. If my car tears up, I can take it down there and he'll fix it. Unbelievably, he can find things about a car that nobody else can find.

Bige R. Warren, Barbourville, November 20, 2008

SLOW-LEARNING GIRL

One of the little girls I had come from another school, and the teacher there told me, said, "You need to worry about her. She can't learn. She can't read, so you just won't be able to teach her; there's something wrong with her."

I took this little girl under my wing and it was hard, but by the end of the year I had her recognizing her letters, her sounds, and the numbers, but she still wasn't reading.

The next year I started teaching her to read, and within two years I had her reading. She was really a slow, slow little girl, and her mother and daddy were slow.

Perhaps I shouldn't have done that with her because I'm sure I neglected some of the other kids by doing that. But I did what I thought was best at the time.

Georgia Lloyd, Barbourville, November 21, 2008

PLAYING SCHOOL

I taught at Glenview in Green County where I had only ten children. I'd pick up some of them and haul them to school because their parents asked me to. There was a guy in the neighborhood who drove his "bucket lid" [pretend automobile] and he'd come to school. While coming, he'd pretend to be playing his radio. He was kind of mentally off, but his parents never had made him go to school. They called him Joker.

Well, I was about half afraid of him, and I told an eighth-grade boy, "I am just afraid of him," and he said, "Miss Ward, he won't hurt you. Just, just, just don't say anything when he comes around the school building. Just ignore him, and he'll quit."

Well, he did quit, then he'd wait for us to come out for recess and he'd play with us. He just loved going to school, and I know they could have sent him to school years ago and he would have learned.

Joyce Williams Ward, Campbellsville, December 11, 2008

ISOLATED BOY

I had only one handicapped student for a short time. He did not enter into any activity. He couldn't make the other students understand him. When that happened he was so upset he cried.

Mattie Jo Smith, Benton, March 7, 2009

MENTALLY DISABLED

Back when I had a seriously mentally disabled boy in school, the school nurse came out to examine students' eyes and do other things that nurses did in those days.

She had to be so many feet away from students to test their eyes. She looked at this boy's eyes and told him to take the tape measure over to a certain place. All he did was just look at her. He couldn't even do what she told him.

I also had two more kids in that family. One of them was really intelligent and the other one was okay.

For the next few years we had to keep all students with limited intelligence in the room with the other kids, even when they were not one-room schools. But after they got all the different programs going, those kinds of kids are taken care of.

Betty Garner Williams, Campbellsville, December 11, 2008

CARING

The only slow-learning student I ever had was a girl who couldn't learn, but she was one of the sweetest students I ever had. She was also so very kind. All the other students loved that child and we just catered to her.

Today we just don't have much care for people. I really believe more learning took place in a one-room school than in one that's highly developed.

Helen Raby, Elizabethtown, January 10, 2009

Chapter 11

BEFORE AND AFTER CONSOLIDATION

The closure of one-room schools betokened a significant educational and cultural change for the communities in which they had operated, a change both for good and for ill, according to the teachers who shared their opinions for this book. The superior resources of the modern consolidated school—from textbooks to the latest technological tools—are undeniable, but some teachers argue that emphasis on and mastery of the basics of education have been sacrificed. The bedrock of one-room teaching style—more advanced students participating in teaching beginning students—comes in for praise as a naturally reinforcing review process, while at the same time it highlights a disadvantage of the older system: the difficulty teachers had giving students individual attention. And yet many former teachers also feel that the one-room classroom offered more opportunity for closer personal relationships between teacher and students.

Interestingly, much of the criticism teachers levy against the modern school is, arguably, cultural rather than academic in nature: today's teachers must spend too much time disciplining children rather than teaching them, today's students have too many distractions in the form of electronic diversions, and so on.

In the end, despite the myriad advantages rural school teachers acknowledge exist in modern schools, what these one-room veterans decry most of all is the loss of certain intangible values that seemingly our schools today cannot supply: mutual respect and a sense of community.

ADVANTAGES AND DISADVANTAGES OF ONE-ROOM SCHOOLS

One of the problems in the rural [one-room] schools that I thought we ran into was keeping order, or keeping the other kids busy, while we were conducting a class. See, we had grade 1 through grade 8, and we'd call them up to a recitation bench and they'd do their ten- or fifteen-minute recitation. While they were reciting, the other kids were supposed to be studying.

One of the main values of the one-room school was that younger kids learned from older kids by listening to their recitations, but sometimes they would get involved in nuisance and it would be difficult to keep them from talking. It was a problem to keep order of the kids that were not in the class when you were having a recitation from another class.

When kids were making noises, I'd say, "Now, keep quiet and do your study like you're supposed to do, so as to let these kids in their class recite for me in their class."

It was a constant review process for kids in higher-class grades to listen to kids reciting in lower-class grades. That's one of the advantages, I think, of the rural one-room schools. The younger children would listen to the older children, and the older children would listen to the younger kids, during their recitations.

One of the disadvantages was the fact that teachers didn't have enough time to spend with individual students, because there were so many students, and so many different grade levels, so many different classes, and so many different subjects that you didn't have a lot of time, and you depended on them to do a lot of home studying to get up to date on their assignments. Most of the students indeed did do that.

The grading system back then was like this: an A grade was 94–100, B was 86 through 93, a C was 78 through 85, and on down the line. Most of the students made average grades. Some students were super outstanding, perhaps due to their parents spending more time with them at home. But some children didn't have much parental guidance. They had very poor backgrounds; not much help from home. That was to be expected in a community that had these rural schools.

J. Robert Miller, Rock Bridge, September 18, 2008

One-Room versus City School

I had a good time teaching at White Oak, and the people were really good to me. Everybody out there called me "Miss Billie"—old people, everybody. They were good to me. They come and mowed the yard, and one man would go to the stock market every week. When he would go, he would bring bananas and pass them out to the kids. They were all good to me.

When I taught the sixth grade here in Edmonton, it was harder. I had a big class, and some of the students were twelve years old, and some of them were sixteen. Some of them were pretty feisty. I think it was harder teaching the sixth grade.

After that first year here in Edmonton, I then began teaching first grade, and that's what I've always loved.

My first year at White Oak I started out scared, but I made it alright out there, as they were all fine children.

Billie Sue Blakeman, Edmonton, September 22, 2008

SMART KIDS AT RURAL SCHOOLS

In providing a viewpoint of the quality of rural schools, the heating was bad. They only had potbelly stoves. I also remember that at times I had to furnish pencils and papers to kids if their parents wouldn't get those things for them. However, most of them were able to get what the kids needed, and did.

I remember one boy that had one tablet that he used the whole year. He would write, then draw a line. He didn't waste any spaces on the sheet of paper. [*Laughter*]

The kids were told not to waste paper at home, I know.

I guess kids in modern-day schools have more advantages, but I've always thought we had some very smart kids that came out of rural schools.

I also think that older kids learned from younger kids as they heard them talk and discuss book matters. And the same is true for the younger kids who listened to some of the things older students were talking about.

I remember when I taught at Angely, I took the eighth graders to Edmonton to take their test to go to high school. They all did pretty well, as most of them passed and got to go on to high school. Some of them didn't go on to high school after they finished the eighth grade in a rural school. The teachers would say, "You ought to go to high school," and the student might say, "Well, my daddy said I didn't have to if I don't want to."

Things like that just burned me up.

Virginia Janes, Edmonton, September 22, 2008

Comparison of Schools Then and Now

I think the schools today have so much more to offer children than the one-room schools did. Of course, times are different now, with all the new technology and everything. Back then we didn't have a lot of reference books in the schools to use in looking up things we needed to know. However, we did have geography and history books, but we didn't do much science teaching.

I think there is a lot of advantage today for students, but our students back then knew how to read, and they all knew how to do simple math when they got out of school, and that's more than you can say about a lot of students today. We taught the basic things, and we did a lot of memory work. As a student I could memorize a poem overnight, and then say it at school the next day.

In the one-room schools we also did a lot of recitation, like multiplication tables. I don't know if they even do that in schools now. You learn your 2s, your 4s, your 5s and 6s, and keep going. You could recite 2 times 2 is 4; 3 times 2 is 6, then go on through the 4s up to the 8s and 10s. I don't think they teach that now.

When we were ciphering on Friday afternoons, that was practicing math. For example, two students would go to the board and the teacher would give them a problem, and the one that got the answer first got to stay up there at the board, but the loser would sit down and another student came up.

We also had spelling bees. You'd have two team captains, one on each side, and they would choose which students they wanted on their side. Of course, they knew who the best spellers were, and you'd choose them. Then the teacher would choose words from the spelling books, then give out the words. They would start with easy words, then use words that were harder to spell. If a kid misspelled a word, they had to sit down. When one side got smaller and smaller, and the other side still had a lot of people standing up, they'd win the contest.

Cipherings and spelling bees were great practice events for students.

Betty Jane (Miller) Pence, Franklin, Tenn., September 29, 2008

"Awfully Smart Children"

I taught only in the elementary grades, and it was only third grade during my last several years. That wasn't a one-room school; it was in the town of Russell Springs.

The last two-room school in Russell County was Jabez, and it closed in the late 1960s. Ronnie Sparks was the last teacher there.

After the one-room schools were closed down, I think I was happy because the schools could have better facilities. However, I don't think the kids learned more in the consolidated schools than they did in the one-room schools. I had some awfully smart children in the old rural schools.

Pearl Helm, Russell Springs, January 24, 2009

Respect

I think that in elementary schools a teacher has a chance to teach twenty students somewhere in the same range, from first through the eighth grade. I liked the way my third-grade classes were going. Of course, in schools now it's guns and everything else. Trying to leave God out is partly the cause.

Back then the children respected the teachers, and we respected the children. It just isn't that way today in some cases.

Marguerite Wilson, Leitchfield, October 1, 2008

Old Times versus New Times

A great deal of education was accomplished in those one-room schools, because they spent their time on real study, and there were very little disciplinary problems. Also, the teacher organized things so that every minute was used to students' advantage, and the older ones helped the younger ones in different grades. Another valuable thing about one-room schools is that while younger kids were reciting, the older ones were listening, and the same thing took place while the older kids were reciting. They all learned from each other. I'm thankful that I went to a one-room school.

A great deal was offered back then, but there's much more offered to young people in schools now than there was then. There's so much more material offered to them relative to the quality of learning. There's a great deal offered, but some of it is wasted because of the lack of discipline and ability for teachers to teach. Too much time is spent on records and that sort of thing.

Virginia DeBoe, Eddyville, October 7, 2008

Parental Involvement

One of the things that was hard for me to see was the disappearance of one-room schools. It caused a closeness of the family to be lost. After that they kind of went separate. It seemed like every parent was interested in each child that was present in the one-room school; then when the school was disbanded, that closeness was lost.

As you look back, we know consolidation was progress for the children, because they had many more opportunities, and many more teaching facilities than all we had down there. But the years of the one-room schools were wonderful years. As I look back on each one of the schools where I taught, it is still a great feeling when my former students see me now, and come running up to hug me and speak to me.

Emma Walker, Eddyville, October 7, 2008

Both Good and Bad

You hear that the younger ones learned from the older ones during the one-room school era, but I don't think the old school times are as good as they are today. How could they possibly be? I'm such a fan of lower class sizes. You can get so much more done in smaller classes today than was possible back then when teachers had to divide their times between eight classes.

On the other hand, children in one-room schools were more likely to obey than kids today. But I liked bad boys! I pretty much got a lot of trouble from them because I liked them. I found the kid that had the worst reputation, but I complimented him. He had to live up to that! That's so true because you don't catch flies with vinegar, or whatever it is. You compliment them to make them know that they can do whatever they're supposed to do. Most kids still live up to it. There are a few exceptions, but not many.

Today's schools are better, but I don't approve of what the kids do when they get home today. Instead of doing some household chores, many of them watch television and play video games all too much.

Maryanna Barnes, Frankfort, October 14, 2008

Green Blackboard

At these one-room schools the little kids would learn from the older ones by just seeing the writing, or what was on the blackboard, put there by older students. When they went to other schools, and if they had a new green board there, you made a mistake if you happened to say, "Let me go to the blackboard," because it was a green board there.

I also need to say that at the one-room schools when the young kids were reciting, the older kids often listened to them, thus it was a constant review process.

Mamie Wright, Tompkinsville, October 16, 2008

Future Prospects

When I was teaching at Independence School I had a very bright eighth grader. I'd had her for several years in school, and she was very smart. At the end of the eighth-grade term our superintendent had a test that all eighth graders had to take before they could enter high school.

She was the only one I had in the eighth grade that year. She took the test and made one of the highest grades in the county. She read everything she could get her hands on, including book after book, and she listened to everything that was going on. She was also very good in math, so she just absorbed everything.

The test she took was more like just a general test. It covered everything, all kinds of questions, such as current events, and she scored one of the highest grades in the county, and I was so proud of her.

In comparing her with today's eighth-grade students, I think she would have done well, but she never went on to high school, as that was very typical back then.

Imogene Dick, Monticello, November 7, 2008

Sustained Education

What I think was better about the one-room schools than those today is that the teacher was there all day long with those students, and you could teach all day long. But now you have so many interruptions by different things that cause children to have to be in and out of the classroom, and that is that.

The day is broken up in present times by so many different things. Back then, when you were in a one-room school, you taught all day long from 8:00 in the morning to 4:00 in the afternoon, except for the time you were out for recess. I think they learned as much back then because they didn't have things brought into the schools like we do today. In other words, as far as their basic education was concerned, I think children back then learned as well as they do today, maybe even a little better.

Wanda Humble, Monticello, November 7, 2008

Bigger Isn't Better

I think the one-room experience is a good teaching experience. I don't think bigger is better. I was flabbergasted in having so much to teach. I went home the first two weeks crying and upset because I couldn't teach all those subjects to all those grades.

I finally put a bunch of books on the shelf, and we taught science to everybody, and social studies to everybody. Students would add to it based on whatever was in their books at their level when we'd be having discussions.

When teaching math, the older children would help the younger ones. Nowadays they give it a fancy term and call it cooperative learning. (Even the little kids would hear the older ones reciting, and they would learn a lot from that.) Well, I was doing that way back when! I did that when I began teaching in the city school, too.

Joyce Campbell Buchanan, Barbourville, November 21, 2008

The Teacher Is the Key

When the one-room school died so did I, as far as teaching was concerned. I never taught in consolidated schools. I have worked with children in consolidated schools, but I never taught in any of them.

My opinion is the teacher is the key. If you had a good teacher in a one-room school, you had a wonderful experience. But there was a teacher that was half drunk and never got to school before Monday at noon because he was still drunk, or had a hangover from the time he left on Friday so he could get drunk over the weekend. He never even learned the kids' names.

All that aside, if you had a really good teacher that really loved the kids and worked with them, you have made it. The same type thing was also in the consolidated school. If you have a good teacher who really works with the kids, then you have a good program anywhere you go.

Irma Gall, Barbourville, November 20, 2008

Personal Attention and Play

Even in the one-room school, I felt that children progressed if they had the right leader as their teacher. They progressed at a fast rate, and it was for personal purposes, as everybody knew everybody. I'm a strong believer in small classrooms. I'm not sure I'm a big believer in all the big schools that we have today. I don't think that students have as much personal attention as they have in a small group. You get much of that from a teacher. For instance, they go from one class to another, and students don't get to know what their teachers are really like. And teachers don't get attached to them.

I never gave a six-weeks grade [grade given at end of first grading period] until I knew every student in every class I had, and I had 150 students. I couldn't do it, because how do you grade a child when you don't know what their capabilities are, or where to put them in a class, and how to assist them?

That first grading period was a horrifying thing for me.

In terms of classroom equipment, back then we had nothing in our classroom unless we bought it. During the last fifteen years I worked as a high school teacher, every year they brought me a ream of paper and two or three other things in a little box. Those were my supplies for the year. If I had anything else, I bought it.

In order to improve the school system for grades first through eighth, we need less testing. In the state of Kentucky, no child is left behind. Too much is given along with CATS [Commonwealth Accountability Testing System] test, which needs to be improved somewhat.

My biggest fault with too much testing is that we are making robots out of our children. They don't have any time for free play. Their schedule is so tight that they have to get all these required things in. When I went to school we had books, recess, lunch, and we had fun in between. We also worked hard in between so we could have fun. But what happens now is our children have to line up to get a drink; line up to go to the bathroom; go to lunch and then have to wait until the rest of the students get through eating; and they have to walk down the halls with their hands behind them so they won't touch the pretty walls. Not all schools are this way, but many are. I'm in a lot of schools and I know what's going on.

What worries me very much is that leadership skills are built in free play. You have to let children be leaders. I remember Christmas before last year when my little great-nephew and the other kids came to my house. I had cooked Christmas dinner for them, about thirty. I watched the children all the time. My little nephew is smaller than the rest of them, and all at once he came running through the house yelling, "Come on, kids, let's go here and do this." That was free play. Now, in my training I tell each council, "Look, find some time each day where you can give those children something to look forward to. After lunch let them have free play. I know safety is a concern, but hide somewhere. Put yourself up a fence or something so you can look and see them without them knowing you are watching them. Just let them play.

I find the greatest weakness right now is that our children don't like school like they did, because they never have anything to look forward to during the day. I stress that point constantly to teachers and others when I travel around the various counties in this part of the state.

As indicated, learning has to be fun.

Daphne H. Goodin, Barbourville, November 21, 2008

Sad Loss

It broke my heart when I heard that one-room schools were to be closed for good. Teaching in those schools were the happiest days of my life, so I sure hated to see them go. I don't care what people say; there was more discipline back then. The kids loved their teachers. It was completely different back then compared to what it is today.

I think kids back then learned just as much, if not more, in those one-room schools than they do right now. Kids were listening when you were teaching other classes, and they would pick up on that. Thus it was a learning process for everyone in the classroom.

I had a lot of girls that went on to make wonderful teachers. They were intelligent, smart, and would pick up on everything. They'd get their work finished and I'd call them back to show them what I wanted them to do, and they did just as well as I did. They were wonderful teachers, but few of them became formal teachers later on in life.

Georgia Lloyd, Barbourville, November 21, 2008

COMMUNITY PRIDE

When I heard one-room schools were going to be closed down for good, it just did something to me inside. To me, something good was going to be taken away. Those little one-room schools provided community participation and community pride because people really liked their school.

Kids in schools today probably learn more than kids did back in one-room schools because of technology and everything. And back then I never did assign a lot of homework. But today, that's just the way of getting the parents to do the kids' work, and that really tore some of them up, especially when they started having this new math, because they couldn't do it.

I always liked to help with homework when classes were finished, especially if you had time to go around and help them, and see if they were doing it right.

Overall, I feel that the school systems today are better than they were back in the one-room school era. However, the teachers today are not respected by the kids like they were back then. We don't have any discipline whatsoever anymore. The teachers and principal can't do anything but expel a student. And if you send them home, you have to send a homebound teacher to them if they are out for anytime at all.

Pat McDonald, Barbourville, November 21, 2008

MIXED FEELINGS

I guess I had mixed feelings when I heard that one-room schools were to be closed down. There was some good in the one-room school system, but they didn't have many materials to work with like kids do today. I feel that made the teachers back then work harder in things that the teacher should have worked harder at. Today they have all these materials that keep the kids busy and hold their attention, but I don't know if there's any difference in the learning process.

One of today's problems is that kids go home, and instead of doing much homework, they watch television and play video games. Many of today's TV programs are not fit to watch.

I still sub teach now and then, and to keep kids busy today a lot of times they'll put on a little cartoon movie, which is fun to watch, but doesn't teach much to the kids watching it. However, they may learn about how to get along and interact with other kids, and maybe learn that there's a quiet time and a not so quiet time.

Laura Agnes Townsley Stacy, Barbourville, November 21, 2008

Good Step Forward

I felt good about it when I heard that one-room schools were to be closed. It was a good step forward in the educational process. My dad and I worked hard to get consolidation at Red Cross, and I went around with him to other schools where he made speeches about consolidation, and took petitions from parents. Of course, there were some people who were opposed to consolidation, but the majority wanted it.

Virginia Galloway, Merry Oaks, December 3, 2008

Gone Are the Good Old Days

One-room schools in Edmonson County included Steep Hollow, Rocky Hill, Union Light, Grassland, Midway, Straw, Hill Grove, Pleasant Union, Fairview, Vincent, Red Hill, Asphalt, Pig, Segal, Sunfish, Silent Grove, and Van Meter.

It was really sad when the one-room schools were taken out of the community. Sometimes the schoolhouse was used for church worship. The people who lived in a community loved their school and would fight the board of education, hoping to keep their school.

I missed the many friends I made at the one-room school. There are lots of old memories that are lost. We were joined together by manners, customs, and our own opinions. We gained experiences that we still use in everyday life. I didn't want the school to leave a void in the county.

The last one-room school in Edmonson County went out in 1958. I believe that students learned more on an annual basis than today's students because there were eight grades in one-room schools. The good students in the higher grades could help the slow students in the lower grades. This kept everyone's attention as the teacher went from grade 1 to grade 8.

When my mother taught school, sometimes she would have eighty students in one room. Anytime the teacher asked a question to a student, everyone in the room listened to see what the answer was. You didn't have any discipline problems in class. There were some problems while playing games, but that was expected.

Today's schools have A.E. [Academic Expectations]. I believe A.E. is not working because my granddaughter has had a very hard time getting through school. She has eight and one-half days left and gets out at midterm. She couldn't stand school any longer, so she took an extra course during her summer break to finish at midterm.

High school was great days for me, but it's different now.

Michael M. Meredith, Bee Spring, December 7, 2008

Praise for One-Room Schools

I was at a funeral home this weekend and one of the boys I had in school said to me, "You were always my favorite teacher. You were good, you saw that we learned, and we achieved. You can't compare what it was like then with what it is today. We learned more, and we accomplished more in the little one-room school than they are doing today."

I also had his brother in the eighth grade when I was teaching in Greensburg. He came up to me at the funeral home and said, "You were one of my favorites, and I can still make 100 on your English tests." He had been a principal, is now retired, and has two grown children. At the funeral home he brought them over and introduced them to me, saying, "This was one of my very favorite teachers."

I think we accomplished more back then, because we had the cooperation of everybody. When you have thirty-five students ranging from first grade through eighth grade, there is quite a bit of work to be done, and these older students helped teach the younger ones, and they also learned from one another. What you were teaching to one group was listened to by others. So there was a definite advantage to the one-room school system.

Bernadine Shirley Sullivan, Campbellsville, December 11, 2008

The Self-Contained School

When I had my orals for my M.A. in 1960 at Western Kentucky University, Dr. Gordon Wilson asked me, "Have you ever taught in a self-contained school?"

My reply was, "It's the only kind in which I've ever taught." At that time I had taught sixteen years in the one-room school.

In a one-room school you were the janitor (building fires, cleaning away ashes, sweeping the floor, dusting, and doing other menial chores). You were also the phys. ed. teacher. I played with the children during recess involving games like town ball, pitching horseshoes, playing tag, ante over the house, and any other game they could come up with.

Art and music was also introduced, but modestly.

All in all, the curriculum was well rounded without the aid of a special teacher.

To me, the one-room school days were the good ole days.

Bernadine Shirley Sullivan, Campbellsville, December 11, 2008

Better Today

In comparing the one-room school system with present-day schools, I feel that students in modern times learn more than those in one-room schools. I feel this way because the one-room schools were too crowded with too many different-age students.

I also feel that teachers were better trained at consolidated schools.

Martha Campbell, Central City, December 13, 2008

Old Times, New Beginnings

Our last one-room schools here in Laurel County were closed at the end of the 1969–70 school year. In 1965 when I moved to the central office we had fourteen one- and two-room schools still operating. They had served well in their day, but that day had passed.

Here is a story to illustrate that point. The Council of Southern Mountains, located in Berea, had collected a lot of donated books. A huge amount of them had been given to the Laurel County System with the expressed desire that they be given to the one- and two-room schools. The system owned an old pickup truck bought from military surplus.

One of my first jobs as a supervisor in 1965 was to distribute these books to the fourteen schools, most of which were located on gravel or dirt roads. The worn steering mechanism on the old truck made it difficult to stay in the road. The books had been stored in an old building donated to the system by the Forestry Service and it contained no heating or cooling systems. Some of the books were boxed up in old military footlockers. Others were thrown in a heap.

I took a blue air force footlocker full of books to Whitson, a one-room school on the west side of the county. After I got them all distributed, a representative of the council came to Laurel County, desiring to visit the schools to see how the books were being utilized.

When we got to Whitson they had a substitute teacher that day. We didn't see any of his books, and she (the teacher) had no idea as to where they had gone. However, we noticed a big blue patch on the front door. The gentleman then said, "Well, at least the *box* was useful."

Laurel County's last twelve one- and two-room schools were finally closed in 1970 as part of a giant reorganization. The London and Laurel County school systems agreed to merge and to build a large senior high school to serve the entire county.

The existing high schools became junior highs, and the small schools' students were brought into the existing consolidated elementary schools. The system later built a second high school and changed to four-year high schools and middle schools. Today our school facilities are among the best in the state.

I felt like it was a step forward when our one-room schools closed. However, I recognized that in days gone by they had served the communities well. It is impossible to really compare the annual amount of learning that took place in one-room schools to that in a modern consolidated school, due to the fact that society has changed even more than the schools. Some of the changes have been good, and some bad. Today there is so much communication and information readily available outside the school. Also, we also recognize that learning is a life-long process. What happens is good in many ways, but change is happening so fast that schools struggle to keep up. Today's students are often more proficient in utilizing technology than their teachers.

The authors of KERA [Kentucky Education Reform Act] recognized that there was value in the approach of the one-room school when they created the primary unit. However, the one-room school simply could not exist today. It could not provide all the services and rights that students and parents have come to expect.

The latter point is illustrated by a story that went around the county when the system began operating a Head Start program. According to the story, a little boy fell on the steps at his school. His teacher helped him up and said, "Don't cry, honey."

The little boy replied, "Cry, hell! I'm going to sue."

We live in a brave new world!

Grover C. Garland, London, December 26, 2008

Old Days versus Present Times

I introduced the students to 16 mm movies and reel-to-reel tape recorders. For them to see a movie and hear the voice on a tape recorder was a new experience. This newfangled technology was state of the art at that time in history.

The one-room school was a rewarding experience for me and I achieved things far beyond my expectations.

The students were very respectful and caused no problems because the parents always said, "If you have a problem let us know." The only absences were sickness, and when the parents set, housed, or stripped tobacco. Some of the older students stayed home to help.

When I moved to a consolidated school with one grade, I felt bad upon receiving my check for teaching just one grade for the same money as that of teaching all eight grades.

In conclusion, let me say that I was concerned for the future of these students in the one-room school. Most were eventually moved to better-equipped schools. Many moved out of the area, even the state, to find jobs. Some have done better than I have in making a living.

Jimmie Jones, West Liberty, December 29, 2008

Trade-offs

When I heard that one-room schools were to be closed down permanently, I knew that children would have to be transported from the district schools to the consolidated schools. I guess consolidation was possible only when county roads were improved so that kids could be bussed to school.

At first two-year high schools were built, but that didn't work because students needed four-year high schools. They had two-year high schools for one year, then the next year they had four-year high schools.

My parents felt that the closure of one-room schools was a wonderful thing because it stood for progress.

Today children are exposed to many more subjects than they were in the one-room schools. They are educated better in certain subjects, but I have an idea that since history and geography were taught as two different subjects in one-room schools, the kids back then learned more than kids do in present times. As for math I'm not sure, because I learned and taught square root in grade school. We knew there were times table, but they don't teach times table at school now like we used to. Teaching square root is also gone.

In the one-room school it seemed that the older children were protective of the smaller children, and some of the younger and older students played together on the playground. That stood for protection and taking care of the little ones. It was kind of like a family situation because of the age spread.

There were advantages to students back then, and there are advantages to today's students. But times back then were truly wonderful, as students learned to work on their own, and they were helpful to each other.

Anna Smith Collins, Marion, November 20, 2008

Unity

The advantages of neighborhood schools are that they provided social and neighborhood unity, teamwork, and protection. Back then people took care of each other.

I remember being bullied by two boys ganging up on me. Two of the older boys took up for me, telling the bullies what they would do to them if they didn't leave me alone. The bullies got the message.

Hale Murphy, Eddyville, December 31, 2008

Loss to Communities

I had a feeling of sadness when I began to see the one-room schools being changed to consolidation. Having attended and having taught in a one-room school, I was well aware of how it was taking such a vital part out of the individual communities.

Never was I against progress; however, to see small communities stripped of this piece of history caused a great concern in my life. It was during the late 1940s and through the 1950s that this process had its huge impact in Metcalfe County.

In one-room schools there was much to be learned by the younger students as they observed the teaching and learning process of the older students. I know that we cannot discount the fact that the children of today have many more materials and many more opportunities to learn than could be provided to children in one-room school settings, but neither did one-room school students have the distractions of today's society.

I am so thankful for being blessed with the opportunity to teach in a one-room school.

Nell S. Eaton, Glasgow, January 8, 2009

No Respect Today

Children in my age went to a one-room school. We didn't have many places to go except to church and school. I feel like those schools have given the world something that schools today can't do. Today's schoolchildren are very unfortunate. They are born to people that don't care for them; parents are separated, and the child becomes really belligerent. Today's children just don't have any respect. I substituted for a long time, but I don't think I could put up with what they are doing now.

Helen Raby, Elizabethtown, January 10, 2009

Voice of Experience

For eighteen years I was affiliated with one-room schools, nine years as a teacher and nine years as a personnel worker. In many rural areas the school was the hub of community activities, such as meetings, bridal and baby showers, and church services.

A dedicated teacher with good management skills and a reasonable pupil load could do a good job. Planning for each grade level was hard and required much time and effort. There was a family-like atmosphere where children learned to care for each other. The young ones learned a great deal by listening to the classes of the upper-grade children.

However, there were adverse conditions not conducive to good educational development. The school terms for the one-room schools were only seven months, although the independent schools had nine-month terms. That was hard for me to understand.

Conditions for the teacher were difficult. In addition to teaching duties, other tasks were overwhelming. The teacher was responsible for the cleaning, heating, play activities, lunch period, and the sick children. There was no electricity and no telephone in any of the one-room schools. Any wonder why the teacher became discouraged?

There was no job security for teachers. They were transferred or, in some instances, dismissed without any consultation explaining why. A few teachers, with a lackadaisical attitude, could be very lax in their duties. There was very little supervision of the teacher or the job they performed. The one-room teachers felt isolated and very much alone.

In 1956 the Greenup Board of Education implemented a plan for consolidation. Five elementary centers would be built and all one-room schools would be closed. Though I had many happy memories about one-room schools, no one was happier than I to see them replaced by a system that provided better educational opportunities for the children of Greenup County.

Vera Virgin, Greenup, January 21, 2009

STUDENTS TAUGHT STUDENTS

I was disappointed when one-room schools were closed down. To me, since there were fewer students in each class, I could do a better job by working one-on-one. One of the truly important things about teaching in one-room schools is that students in lower grades listened to those in the upper grades. The same thing happened when those in the upper grades listened to recitations about different subjects made by students in younger classes; it was a constant review process for the older ones.

One of the best things that happened after consolidation was that buses began running and students could ride to school, not walk.

Dorothy Booker, Marion, January 23, 2009

TECHNOLOGY

If I should go into a classroom today, after retirement of thirty-three years, I am sure that I would feel like the proverbial bull in a China closet, seeing laptops, computers, DVDs, and I would hope to see eager and expectant children's faces. I would be glad to see them being taught to adapt to their technical world. At the same moment, I remembered one of my one-room schools and decided that they had played an important step in being the first rung in the ladder of technology. For the time period in our history, one-room schools taught practical and even cultural advantages and needs to rural communities.

I am proud and glad of my three years in one-room schools and feel that they contributed a large role to the education world.

Maurine Everley Grant, Owensboro, February 4, 2009

DEDICATION

The most poignant thing I can remember about my two years in a one-room school was the eagerness of the students to learn, and how excited they became over discovering a new fact and putting it together with something they already knew.

Education has gained a lot through the years, and has better methods of teaching maybe, and certainly more teaching assets. But the dedication and the enthusiasm of the teachers of the one-room school period was something to be admired, and something I don't think we'll ever get back to.

Betty Jo Arnett Lykins, Salyersville, February 1, 2009

INTERRUPTIONS

There were some good things that came from one-room schools. There were writing lessons, spelling lessons, and multiplication tables that had to be learned. In written work, if a word was misspelled it was counted wrong. Today one can hardly read some written works due to handwriting and spelling. This is from high school and college students, who put too much dependence on computers. They don't have to memorize the multiplication tables the way I did, nor how I taught. There is much, much more for students to learn these days, so writing, spelling, and math are neglected. In my latest years of teaching, students were pulled away from my classroom for music, remedial math, reading, and other things.

I had a student who nearly failed math because her mother wanted her to take violin lessons and miss math class. There are a lot of interruptions like this in today's classrooms. The classroom teacher has too much to do for so many interruptions.

I never had a student in the one-room school that needed remedial work. It seems that in the last few years the cases have multiplied.

I only taught for two years in one-room schools, but I enjoyed every minute of it. Today, when I go to the annual banquet at Rineyville, I see some of my students. One lives in California, one in Louisville, and some in Rineyville and Elizabethtown. It brings back old memories when I see them.

Grace W. McGaughey, Lexington, January 29, 2009

Better Education

I was elated when I heard that one-room schools were to be closed. I then felt that students would get a better education because teachers were better educated and had more to offer their students. I don't remember exactly when that occurred.

There are so many resources now available in a larger school, like a library, cafeteria, gym, etc. I have also found teachers to be better prepared for specific grade levels.

In terms of behavior, however, students were much better behaved in the smaller one-room school environment than in today's schools.

Emogene A. Browning, Louisville, January 23, 2009

Sorry to Leave

After teaching at Davis Bend, I also fell in love with the kids at Cannon, a two-room school. My husband would get them when I got through with them. We had them for eight years. I taught the first four grades, and my husband taught the upper four grades, and boy, we had a pack of them too! There were over a hundred of them one year. The superintendent, Mr. Lay, came out to talk with us and we were just turning out for recess. He said, "I can't believe that you all have this many children. How in the world do you discipline them?"

My husband started the first ball team that any school there ever had. He put up a goal post, and bought uniforms for the boys. I had a group of cheerleaders that I bought some cheerleader outfits for them. We taught those children a completely different lifestyle than what they had been living.

We were there five years, and neither of us wanted to leave. However, the county was closing the school, as they were consolidating all Knox County schools.

Georgia Lloyd, Barbourville, November 21, 2008

Yesterday and Today

Older students were very helpful. The blackboard was used a lot. Many who were good in penmanship would copy things on the board for me. It was a big happy family.

In good weather several students rode their bicycles to school. One young boy who lived nearby rode his tricycle! Many children walked to school. How that differs today! Children and parents respected the teacher's opinions and methods. Many came to school without the knowledge of things children know today. Back then there were no preschool, no kindergarten, no educational television programs. I think the one-room schools' success relates to the attitudes of people in those days.

I retired in 1986 after teaching five years in one-room schools and the remaining twenty-five years in consolidated schools at the junior high level. Only a teacher knows the amount of work and caring it takes. I loved it all!

Patricia Gibson, Greenup, April 11, 2009

Chapter 12

Home Life of Students

Many rural students came from desperately poor families. Families were frequently large, and at times there was not enough food to go around. Some families were also what we in modern terms would call dysfunctional, as one or two stories below graphically illustrate.

It is perhaps in the nature of things that teachers would remember and talk about the failures rather than the successes in discussing this topic, but other stories throughout this collection, as well as the last one given here, show that regardless of hard times, love and support among families also abounded.

Caring for Poor Kids

The kids always brought their lunch meal from home, and I had one family in which the mother had died. Their daddy was raising their four children, and these children would come to school in the mornings, then they would go home. A lot of days they wouldn't come back during the afternoon. They lived a long way from school and had to walk to and from school. They didn't come back because they hadn't had anything to eat.

Well, I took some things and would give them food, but I didn't have a lot either back then. I was working hard to get by. But those kids have all come along okay. Two of them were girls, and those two girls are the ones that organize our reunion every year.

Zona Royse, Columbia, October 4, 2008

Welfare Family Students

I had one family here in Knox County that had twenty-two children, and I had eleven of them in school. They lived in a three-room house—two log rooms and a lean-to on the back. Not all of those twenty-two kids were at home, but about eighteen of them were there at home. They were short of money and everything, but they were on welfare. So they almost had more money than anybody else. Welfare made sure they had clothes.

Eight to fifteen children was a common thing for families back then. I had four or five children from the same home.

Irma Gall, Barbourville, November 20, 2008

Poor Lunch

Students would bring biscuit sandwiches, of course, and fried eggs, boiled eggs, fried chicken, cookies, sausage, and cake. Whatever they had at home, they'd make some of it into sandwiches and bring it to school.

One time this neighbor boy came to our house and was going to ride with my brother to high school. Somehow something happened to his lunch. They had wrapped it in newspaper, so to take care of it and not let it ruin, my mother took it inside and unwrapped it. She said it was just peanut butter and crackers—several of those, but that was all. She said that she wanted to put a biscuit and ham in it, but didn't dare do it because it might have been insulting. So she just wrapped his peanut butter and crackers back up.

Virginia DeBoe, Eddyville, October 7, 2008

Thievery Forgiven

At Miller's Creek School many children brought something such as a snack for first recess or last recess. Several children had a long walk to and from school. If I remember, when I was in first or second grade I had saved an apple one time for the last recess. When I looked for my apple at my desk and didn't find it, I told the teacher that the boy next to me had my apple.

He didn't deny that he had it, but the teacher did nothing, not even to scolding the boy. He was a member of one of the two poorest families in the community. Our teacher and families were very good at teaching us morals and compassion for others.

After I grew up I understood more and admired the teacher, while sympathizing with the boy. The teacher knew that Tom had little or nothing to eat, and I didn't need the apple, for if I did I could always get more.

Pauline Keene Looney, Pikeville, December 8, 2008

Grandfather's Contribution

I remember that Grandfather would get up from the table after all family members had finished eating lunch. He would then pick up the kettle of beans and one containing potatoes, along with an extra pan of cornbread. He would wrap the cornbread in a cloth, put it in a flour sack, put the handle, or bail, of each kettle over his arm and prepare to leave the house.

With these food items in his hands, he would leave the house and get on his mule or horse. My grandmother would tell him that he was taking the family's supper. She always cooked both meals while the stove was hot.

After she said that to him, Grandfather told her that one or two families had not had enough food for lunch or dinner. The little boy, Tom, that stole my apple was one of these families Grandfather took food to.

I fully understood why my grandfather did that.

Pauline Keene Looney, Pikeville, December 8, 2008

Little Girl without Shoes

A story that comes to mind is about this little girl whose name I won't call. It was cold weather, windy and rainy in November, and she was still barefooted. I didn't know what to do for her, but I had her to put her foot on a piece of paper, and I drew an outline of her foot onto the paper. . . .

My uncle Bill had two dry goods stores on the square. I took the sheet of paper with this little girl's footprint to Uncle Bill, and he looked at it and knew right off what size shoes she needed. So I bought her a pair of shoes and took them to her. I said to her, "Now, [name omitted], you take care of these. Don't you be running and jumping up and down in mud holes."

She told me that she wouldn't, but in just a few days later I was riding in the taxi going home, and there she was running along and jumping in every mud hole. She was hitting them all! [*Laughter*]

She is also the only one that never had any food for lunch. Mama would always fix an extra sandwich or two, cookies, and apples and things, so I could give this girl something to eat.

Her parents were very poor. When I visited their home, there were several of her family members there, and I thought this is what chickens live in. It was pitiful. One of [name omitted]'s sisters had cut her foot real bad one time, so I took some fruit and other stuff when I went to visit them. I was in shock. I couldn't believe that a house full of people could live like that.

I don't guess she ever went to the doctor.

Billie Sue Blakeman, Edmonton, September 22, 2008

Pregnant Student

One day one of the girls in the eighth grade was absent. She was a real sweet, pitiful girl, but she had a good personality. I asked, "Where's Marie today?"

She also had a brother in school there. They looked to be about two years apart, but they both were in the same grade. He said that Marie is sick. So I passed by her house on my way from school and stopped to see her.

The door to their house was open, so I looked in. I said, "Are you in there, Marie?"

She said, "Yeah, I'm over here," and there was a bed back over there.

I said, "Honey, what's wrong?"

She said, "Miss Lloyd, I'm pregnant."

I said, "Oh, gosh, do you know who is the daddy?"

She said, "Yeah, right over there he sits," and that was her brother!

He said, "Yeah, I got her pregnant, and I'll get you that way, too, if you'll come over here."

Well, I got out of there. I told my husband, and he said, "I don't want you to go back."

I said, "I'll go back until Christmas, then I'll go back to college. I can't leave them without a teacher."

Georgia Lloyd, Barbourville, November 21, 2008

DYSFUNCTIONAL FAMILIES

I had students that were more than slow learners. In one instance I had students that came from a family and they were so emotionally upset when they came to school. I had four or five students from one family that were so upset with each other and with their parents that they couldn't begin to learn.

I had to do a lot of psychological quieting down. That type problem was too prevalent. In one creek school I had trouble with moonshine whenever there was a runoff of moonshine whiskey. A lot of the men went out there and got drunk, then came home and beat their families and the women went up the hill.

I remember one instance in which the children often left their house with their mother that took the children out and slept in a whole row of junk cars along the creek. The kids slept out there because their father and mother were quarreling with each other.

So I had a lot of instances like that when dysfunctional families couldn't get along with each other.

Irma Gall, Barbourville, November 20, 2008

DESPERATELY POOR

The superintendent sent me to teach at a school located in a holler [hollow], one mile off the road that led to an old coal mining community. The school was held in a church in that community. My husband would drop me off there, and I'd walk about a mile up to the school. He had two other teachers that rode with him and he was taking them to their schools. He didn't have time to take me all the way up there.

The children weren't clean, and there was odor in the school and church when they would come in. In fact I had talked with some of the little girls that had stains on the back of their dresses to tell them what they needed to do, and how they needed to clean themselves up.

I had one little boy that was the most pitiful thing I've ever seen. So that afternoon I went into town and bought clothing for him, then gave them to him the next day. I said to him, "When you go home tonight, wash really good and take a bath." I didn't know if they had a bathtub or not. I went on to say, "Put these clothes on."

He said, "Okay."

The next day he came back in the same old clothes. I said, "Where's the clothes I bought you?"

He said, "I traded them for a piece of meat and bread."

Georgia Lloyd, Barbourville, November 21, 2008

Bad Home Lives

There were five boys that brought homebrew to school and hid it in the boys' toilet. One of the girls slipped and told me. I brought the boys inside, talked to them in earnest, then I proceeded to give them spankings. That's one thing they remember.

It did not deter some of them, as they were drinkers in later life, but some did not imbibe. Whether that was a cause of their not drinking, I don't know.

There's another memorable time when a fourth- or fifth-grade boy was supposed to be studying his spelling. From the front of the room, having lower grade classes, I called the child's name and said, "You'd better be studying your spelling."

Color was gone from his face, and God was guiding me, as I said nothing else. At recess one of the siblings lifted his shirt and I saw marks made by a blacksnake whip.

I cringe to think this today. It taught me that you never know the circumstances of children before and after school.

Betty Holmes McClendon, Nancy, January 26, 2009

Compulsory Schooling

One family with four students lived near the school. Those four students went home for lunch each day, after their father allowed them to come to school rather than he go to jail.

Mattie Jo Smith, Benton, March 7, 2009

Family Squabbles

My second year teaching in a one-room school in Carter County was in a school known as Fourmile. It was located at Leon just a few miles from

Grayson, Kentucky. Some great families and students lived in the community. Unfortunately, some families with blood kinship were always in a squabble. As a result, their children had disagreements traveling to and from school. This carried over into the school atmosphere.

Patricia Gibson, Greenup, April 11, 2009

In Loco Parentis

When I was teaching up in Missouri Hollow, there were no cell phones, no telephone, thus no way to call anybody to get help when anyone got hurt at school. Well, I had this little girl that was walking down the aisle and hung her foot in the leg of the school bench. She fell and broke her arm right there in the aisle.

Of course, there were forty-some students there at school, so I thought, "What am I going to do?" There was no way I could get help, so all I could do was send the children home.

This girl's mother and father were older parents, and they had no vehicle or anything to take this child to the doctor. Dr. McHargue, who is now deceased, was one of the doctors here in Monticello, and he was their family doctor.

So I sent the children home but told one of the boys that lived close by to go tell the girl's mother and father I was taking her on to the doctor to get her arm set, and for them to come and pick her up later.

I took her on down to Dr. McHargue and paid him for getting her arm set. Believe it or not, the girl's parents never did come to pick her up. Of course, they didn't have a vehicle, so I don't know whether or not they could get someone to bring them. Anyway, Dr. McHargue said he knew where they lived and said to me, "I'll take her home for you."

He took her to her home, and I paid him for setting her arm, but I never did get a dime for it. They were supposed to pay me back, but they never did.

Wanda Humble, Monticello, November 7, 2008

Vicious Cycle

One time one of the kids was asked what he planned to do when he grew up. He said he "planned to draw."

Someone said, "Oh, you want to be an artist?"

He said, "No, I want to draw a check!" [*Laughter*]
That's the kind of culture that just keeps on going.

Velois S. Fitts, Winchester, as told to Deborah Evans Colburn,
March 17, 2009

Like Father, Like Son

I had this little boy as a student, and his father was a bootlegger in the Mt. Pisgah community. He was in the second grade, but was eleven years old. Most of the students then didn't get to come to high school from way out there, as there was no way for them to travel to get to high school. So they just stayed at home and continued to go on to a one-room school.

This eleven-year-old boy came to school one day and he was drunk. He was as wild as anything you've ever seen. He was cursing, mistreating other students, and doing everything. I finally found out what was wrong with him when I smelled whiskey on his breath. I questioned him about it, and he said, "Yes," he had been drinking that morning. Well, I sent him home.

I looked in the record book to make sure how old he was, and he was eleven.

Wanda Humble, Monticello, November 7, 2008

Death in the Family

You don't know what all I went through [as a new teacher]—things I never dreamed of. It was all new to me. One Monday morning I went to school, and there were the worst odors I've ever smelled when I passed by a house. I didn't say anything about it at school, and we went on and had class that day.

The next day you could smell it all the way up to the schoolhouse. I said to the kids, "Do you know what that odor is? What is it?"

This little boy said, "My daddy; that's my daddy. He died Friday night. He got his paycheck and ate a whole hog's head, and he died."

I said, "Is he still in the house?"

"Yep. We slept with him, and he was so hard and cold that we pushed him out of the bed."

Well, I came into town and I went to Aunt Mary, a health nurse who lived across the street from me. I told her there was a dead body in a house near where I was teaching.

So they went up there and got the body. The men in the community built a box and dug a grave. I took my students all up there when they buried him. They just put him in a box, dropped him down in the grave and covered him up, and his own son said, "There he goes in that hole," and just laughed. There wasn't a song; there wasn't a prayer; there wasn't anything.

There were only three more days until Christmas, and it was the hardest thing in the world for me to go to school those three days. But I quit teaching there at Christmas, and Mr. Lay said that he didn't blame me.

Georgia Lloyd, Barbourville, November 21, 2008

Soot Rabbits

Davis Bend here in Knox County was a community where everybody knew everybody, everybody helped everybody; there was no animosity. There was one family that moved in while I was there and lived in an old dilapidated shack. Their kids came to school, and they were good looking kids and sweet, but they were dirty.

I didn't know that my other students had given them a nickname till they left. They only stayed for a month or two. They moved because their house wasn't warm enough.

One of the students said, "Well, the soot rabbits moved."

I said, "The what?"

They said, "Soot rabbits moved."

The others nicknamed those kids the soot rabbits because they were dirty. They had come to school with all that soot on them

The other kids really liked them. I tried to get those kids to clean up, but evidentially that house was so cold they had no way to do it.

Georgia Lloyd, Barbourville, November 21, 2008

Smart Family

This small community had about three or four different family names. These families were interested in their children getting an education, so most of the children completed high school, and a high average went on to college or a trade school. Just to mention one family of five kids, four were college educated and one was trained in his field.

Pauline Keene Looney, Pikeville, December 8, 2008

CONCLUSION

The stories and viewpoints contained in these accounts of early school years across the Commonwealth of Kentucky are truly irreplaceable. The storytellers' historically significant descriptive accounts of the one-room school era are heritage landmarks. Thankfully, they have been recorded before these teachers, like so many others of the period, are gone. But they will never be forgotten by the students, other teachers, family, and community members they inspired.

Betty Holmes McClendon, of Nancy, Pulaski County, who told many stories included in this book, wrote the following inspirational essay, "My Philosophy of Education," some years back. Her words express the fundamental missions of education, whether in the one-room era or in our own times.

> If the aim of education is to improve the lives of the children we teach, then we must introduce them to new ideas and concepts in a way which gives meaning to them.
>
> Children need to see relationships between learning and living in order that they understand the necessity for learning. Children in elementary grades need to be given a good general background of all learning in order that they may later choose wisely their area of specialized learning. If a child can read well, he will be able to find any fact he may need to know; thus I feel that teaching skills in reading and locating information is of greater importance than trying to teach him to memorize isolated facts.
>
> An example should be set by teachers for children, as many times they reflect our attitudes and actions. We should guide them in moral learnings, as well as factual learnings from

books. Children should be taught to use the learnings they acquire and apply them to their own everyday experiences.

Just as we give praise to a child for doing good work, we must also give criticism for work which isn't good, in our judgment. . . . We should try to help the child to accept this as a help toward doing better work, rather than making the child feel incapable in doing properly what is to be done.

Biographies of Storytellers

Maryanna Barnes, Frankfort

I was born September 28, 1937, in Irvine, Estill County. I went to West Irvine Elementary School, then graduated from high school in 1954. After that I went to Eastern Kentucky State College one summer and took a physical education class, a class relative to teaching in a rural one-room school, and an English class.

I started teaching in September, and after I began teaching they found out I was only seventeen years old, but they let me continue because my birthday was September 28. I didn't have to quit! That school was a very rural one-room school in Estill County, and its name was Granny Richardson Springs School. That school building is now located on the campus of Eastern Kentucky University.

I taught at Granny Richardson School for two years, taught one year at Station Camp, which was also a one-room school, and then I taught for two years at Pitts Elementary School. The latter was really an interesting experience.

After teaching for five years in these one-room schools, I then taught one year in Ohio, and then I received my degree in one year after I got married. Then I went back to Estill County and taught in a new two-teacher school in West Irvine. I taught fifth grade.

After that my husband got his degree, so we went to Florida where I taught for one year. The students I taught there were Seminole Indians and Cubans, but mostly Indians, as that was their first year off the reservation. That was interesting.

When we came back to Kentucky, I taught two and one-half years at Jenny Rogers School, Danville. And that was really a good experience. After that we came to Frankfort, and I taught third grade for twenty-one years here at Bridgeport.

All total, I taught about thirty-two years.

Norma (Stephenson) (Coffey) Bertram, Monticello

I was born August 17, 1937, in Wayne County when my parents lived in the Parnell community north of Monticello. After completing my elementary years at Parnell, I attended Wayne County High School in Monticello, graduating May 17, 1946. My college work was at Eastern Kentucky State Teachers College (now Eastern Kentucky University), from which I received my B.S. degree in elementary education, 1964.

From just a small child, I knew I wanted to be a teacher. My father, O. B. Stephenson, was a teacher, and my mother stressed God first, then education. I taught with my father at Parnell for three years.

My first college course was a six-week training session at Somerset High School. After school ended each year, we emergency teachers would attend spring and summer terms at a college, so I continued on at Eastern Kentucky. After two years of college credits, students were then certified as teachers.

During World War II, a lot of teachers left the teaching profession to work in factories up north, due to patriotism and/or better pay. This led to a shortage of teachers, especially in the more remote sections of Wayne County.

I retired from teaching in 1986, having taught a total of thirty-seven years. I have a daughter who is a teacher, a nephew [who is also a teacher], and a granddaughter who is studying to be a teacher.

Billie Sue Blakeman, Edmonton

I grew up here in Edmonton, except for a few months as a baby in the mountains, and in Louisville. My dad was Lawrence Lee Isenberg, and my mother was Magdalene Wilson. My mother was born on her sister's birthday, who was six years old at that time. Believe it or not, my grandmother (their mother) died on their birthday.

After graduating from high school, I went two years to Lindsey-Wilson College, a junior college back then. After I went there, I finished at Western in Bowling Green. I majored in elementary education. I received my degree from Western during the summer of 1953 because I had to work my way through school. I taught during the year, went to school during the summer, and also went to school on Saturday.

To get to Western I rode an old school bus every Saturday until I got my degree. . . . The bus didn't cost us anything, because the county provided the bus service. However, it was rough having to ride it, because I would be out on a date until 1:00 or 2:00 in the morning, then I had to get on that bus really early. We lived right close on the square, and a lot of time somebody on the bus would come knock on the door and say, "We're waiting on you; come on."

When that happened I'd throw my clothes on and tear out the door. Well, one time they went off and left me, so we jumped in the car and Mama took us to Glasgow, and we were standing there waiting for the bus to pull up when they got to Glasgow.

Dorothy Booker, Marion

I was born November 11, 1918, in Caldwell County. I graduated from Flat Rock High School in Fredonia, 1936. After I received an emergency certificate from Murray State College in 1943, I taught at Enon School, Caldwell County, 1943–44, then at Creswell, 1944–46, and at Piney Fork School, Crittenden County, 1948–53. All of these were one-room schools. I also taught four years at Mattoon, two years at Union with three teachers, then I taught at Fohs Hall.

I attended Murray State College and received a B.S. degree in 1956, a master's degree, 1962, then did additional college work, also at Murray, 1966–68.

My husband, Clinton Booker, and I are parents of a son, Jimmie, and two daughters, Joanne and Judy. Both daughters are teachers.

I taught school for thirty-eight years in Caldwell and Crittenden counties, and also served as librarian in Crittenden County.

Emogene A. Browning, Louisville
    The oldest of ten children, I was born August 29, 1924, in Millard, Kentucky. During my school years, I attended McAndrews Elementary School in McAndrews, Kentucky, then graduated from Belfry High School in 1941. I attended Pikeville Junior College, then enrolled at Nazareth College, Louisville, from which I obtained a B.S. degree.
    I taught at Sharondale Elementary, Stone Elementary, and Aflex Elementary for a total of ten years in Pike County. I later taught at Rockford Lane Elementary and Crums Lane Elementary, both of which are in Louisville. I retired from Jefferson County Public Schools in 1982 after a total of twenty-eight years. I am proud to say that I was a teacher in Kentucky for thirty-eight years.
    I married Roy C. Browning Sr. November 26, 1947, and we had one son, R. Clifford Browning Jr., who retired after thirty-three years of teaching and serving as a principal, and our daughter-in-law retired from teaching after twenty-nine years of service.

Joyce Campbell Buchanan, Barbourville
    I was born May 25, 1940, in Coalport, Knox County. I attended Artemus Elementary School through the eighth grade. Artemus also had a high school at that time, and I went there my first high school year. I graduated from Knox Central High School, 1957, then enrolled at Union College that fall. I graduated from Union four years later, with a major in elementary education. I received my master's degree in education from Union College in 1980.
    I had to borrow a ride to college when I was a freshman since I wasn't driving yet. The superintendent of Knox County Schools was in this car with my friend that was taking me home. He asked me what I was going to do when I got through college, and I said, "I guess I'll be a secretary."
    He said, "Well, Joyce, you know there's not many secretary jobs in this area."
    I got to thinking about what he said, then decided that I would follow my mother's steps and be a teacher.
    My mother was a two-room school teacher who taught at Wheeler, which was above Coalport and Brush Creek. I know she had to walk from the main road a long distance from home to and from the school. She taught at Artemus Elementary School for twenty-seven years. She had varicose vein surgery and a blood clot that went into her lungs. She died during her thirtieth year of teaching. Both of my children are also educators. . . .
    Although it is not really true, as far as I'm concerned, while teaching I was the superintendent, the principal, the teacher, the janitor, and the cook!!

Martha Campbell, Central City
    I was born October 5, 1914, in Muhlenberg County. I graduated from Greenville High School in 1932. Back then it was not necessary for one-room school teachers to go to college. I did, however, attend Bethel College in Hopkinsville for one year, but I did not continue my college education because I felt it was too expensive for my parents.
    I decided to become a teacher because I needed a job and thought teaching would be interesting. My first teaching job was at Sharon School, located southwest of Greenville. The road from Greenville to Hopkinsville was being built that year. In order to get to Sharon, I drove my husband's Ford Roadster, but when the road was muddy I rode a horse.

The way I got my first teaching job was the result of my dad talking to a trustee about it. What happened is that the regular teacher had taken off for one year, so I got her job. However, she came back the following year and replaced me.

When I first started to teach, I was still living with my parents, located about three miles from the school. When my husband and I got married October 6, 1934, we moved into his parents' house, located in the Pleasant Hill community east of Greenville. From that new home it was quite a trip for me to make every day to get to school, especially on horseback. Sometimes I even stopped at my parents' house to spend the night.

Shelby Jean Caudill, Madisonville

A native of Letcher County, I was born October 30, 1936. My parents, Clifton (an author) and Ruby Haynes Caudill, who lived in a log cabin, had five children, three boys and two girls, all of whom were delivered by midwives. I graduated from Stuart Robinson High School, May 1956, then attended Eastern Kentucky University for two years. I taught for three years at Bull Creek, a one-room school in Letcher County.

In December 1957, during Christmas break, I married my high school sweetheart, Lee Caudill, who had just returned from a three-year stay in Germany with the U.S. Army. Lee was stationed at Ft. Knox and we newlyweds saw each other only once a month during the first eight months of our marriage. Lee had to return to Germany in September 1959, and this time I joined him in Munich just before Christmas that same year. Our son, Robert Lee, was born at the Army Hospital in Munich, 1961, and the three of us eventually returned to Kentucky in 1964.

I worked for nine years in two official positions at Outwood, while taking night and summer classes at Murray State University, from which I graduated with a bachelor of science degree, 1970; master of arts in education, 1973, and Rank 1, 1977. I eventually served for twenty years as guidance counselor for all grades K–12 at Dawson Springs, Hopkins County, and retired in December 1994.

Anna Smith Collins, Marion

My older sister had gone to a business college in Evansville, Indiana. Three years after I graduated from high school, my father wanted to send me to Evansville for a business education. I said, "Daddy, I don't want to go that way; I'd rather be a teacher."

A few days later, one morning at breakfast he gave me a check and said, "You'd better go to town and get this check cashed and buy you a new hat and two or three new dresses, some pretty shoes, hose, etc., because you'll be going to Bowling Green in the morning."

My dear mother said, "Edgar, she cannot go. She's only seventeen, but not quite seventeen and a half years old. That child cannot go that far away from home."

Daddy prevailed, and at 10:00 the next morning I caught a train to Bowling Green. I arrived in Bowling Green at 10:00 that night.

This little young woman didn't know where she was going, but there in Bowling Green I met some people from Crittenden County. They were sisters to the superintendent of schools and we became roommates. During the second semester at Western, I worked in the dining room for my board, and I did chores at the office in the executive building. I picked up ten cents, fifteen cents, or a quarter if I could as payment for each hour of work. That helped pay for things I needed there at church.

At the end of the semester you could sell your books and get a small percentage of their value back. In fact, you could buy used books.

I graduated from Western in 1939 with an A B. degree, then from Murray State with a master's degree in later years. I also attended Evansville College, and Jefferson College in Missouri.

I taught in one-room schools for a total of three years, many years in grades 1 through 12, and six years as supervisor of instruction in Crittenden County after consolidation. All total, I taught and served for forty-four years.

James W. Crabb, Bowling Green

James Wade Crabb was born January 24, 1858, in Warren County. . . . He married Annie Arbuckle and they parented three boys.

Beginning in 1874, Crabb taught one-room schools in Butler County (three), Hardin County (one), Edmonson County (one), Ohio County (one), Barren County (one), and Warren County (thirteen). He taught at Western Kentucky State College and also served as dean until 1926. He was clerk in the Warren County Superintendent's office, 1926–27.

All total, Crabb spent fifty-five years in teaching and other school work, then retired at age seventy-two. In his latter years he wrote, "I feel in the main I did my best consistently and perhaps did some good in the world. Over a hundred of my former pupils have gone far beyond me in an educational way, yet there is a small number out of probably 3,000 boys and girls who attended my schools."

James W. Crabb died May 22, 1948, and was buried in the Sand Hill Cemetery.

The bulk of this information was derived from Kentucky Explorer, *April 2003*

Kolema Stearns Davis, Taylorsville

I was born in Clinton County, Kentucky, 1926. I began my school days at Indian Creek one-room school, from which I graduated in 1939, then graduated from Clinton County High School, 1943. I attended college at Lindsey-Wilson, Columbia, from which I received an emergency teaching certificate six weeks later. I was only seventeen years old at that time, but the state law said you had to be eighteen before being employed as a teacher. However, I did teach at Willis Creek School, 1944–45. I continued going to Lindsey-Wilson and received my first valid teacher's certificate in 1946.

I attended Western Kentucky State Teachers College during the spring, 1946, then received a B.S. degree in education at Indiana University, 1962, and an M.S. degree in education at Indiana University, Southeast, Jeffersonville, 1972.

In 1961 I taught at John C. Strother Elementary School, Louisville, then during the following six years I taught at Thomas Jefferson Elementary School, Clark County, Indiana. Subsequently, I taught at Silver Creek Junior High School and Stout Elementary School during the next eighteen years. I retired in 1987 after teaching for thirty-two years, six of which were one-room schools in Clinton County.

A lot of my family members were teachers. My dad and two of his sisters, Maude Shearer and Verlie Dickerson, were all teachers. Another of his sisters, Vergie Stearns, had four children, all of whom taught school, and my two sisters, Ramelle Cole and Kate Dowell, taught school. My mother had an aunt, Zula Conner Young, who taught in Georgia and Florida, and Zula's two daughters also taught schools.

Our family has a long line of teachers, and hopefully this tradition will continue throughout the forthcoming generations.

Virginia DeBoe, Eddyville

I was born March 9, 1919, in Madison, Indiana, because there was a hospital there, which is just across the river from Milton, Kentucky, where we lived at that time. Back then there was a ferry across the Ohio River. My mother went across the river early because it was March, and there was still a chance of ice in the river. So, that's why I was born in Madison, but we lived in Trimble County.

My father was Enoch Russell Nowlin, and my mother Ella McIntire Nowlin. My mother went to a one-room school, but I'm not sure about my father, because he grew up in Lawrenceburg, Indiana, but I'm almost positive that he did also.

I personally decided to become a teacher because that was about the only thing available for women then, except for nursing also. In 1938 I went to Western in Bowling Green and just took general classes. It just sort of developed that I leaned toward education, so I obtained the two-year provisional elementary certificate, and I was ready to teach after that. Since then I have done more college work, but that was the way it was at that time.

I didn't teach while my children were very small. So when my last child was born, I knew that I had to go back to college to get my degree then, so I went to Murray State College as a full-time student, and finished there in 1962 with a B.S. degree in elementary education. That fall I began teaching at Nabb School, a one-room school in Caldwell County. I taught there my second year, then moved with my husband to Greensburg in 1942. He taught there as a vocational agriculture teacher.

In 1946 we moved from Greensburg to Taylorsville, then to Eddyville when the schools were consolidated in Lyon County, but I didn't teach until our small kids were all ready to go to school. I then began teaching fifth and sixth grades in the consolidated school in Eddyville. However, there were still a lot of one-room schools in this county.

When my youngest daughter was born, I went back to college at Murray.

All total, I taught three years in one-room schools, one year at Norfork in Trimble County, 1938–39, and two years at Nabb in Caldwell County, 1940–42.

Blanche Demunbrun, Glasgow

I was born in 1907 in the Steep Hollow area in Edmonson County. We lived on a small farm, but my father worked with his older brother building schoolhouses. . . . They built these one-room schoolhouses all across Edmonson County. After my father got through building schoolhouses, he helped to build Lock 6 on the Green River.

I decided to become a teacher when I graduated from Brownsville High School. I enrolled at Western Kentucky State College, and I was also going with Truman Demunbrun, my future husband at that same time. My cousin wanted to go to Western, and I decided I'd go and get a teacher's certificate, because that's what my cousin wanted to do. The two of us went there together. That's when I really got acquainted with Truman.

I got a two-year teacher's certificate to teach. Truman had just graduated from Odgen College, also there in Bowling Green. I think he taught for one year in Muhlenberg County. After that he came to Brownsville and worked awhile in the sheriff's office. Of course, he knew Charlie Whittle, who was president of Odgen College. Truman had already taken a test and passed the bar examination they gave in Frankfort. Upon receipt of that, he didn't have to go to law school. Well, Whittle helped Truman in studying to take the bar exam, so he became a lawyer. He took the last bar exam that they gave in Frankfort. He passed that exam, and we were seeing each other a little at that time.

I became a teacher and taught in one-room schools for two years at Steep Hollow and Temple Hill, then began teaching in a two-room school at Bee Spring in Edmonson County. At Bee Spring, I taught the first-, second-, and third-grade students, and there were sixty-four of them.

When I started teaching, I was paid only sixty dollars per month, each year. And my husband was just starting out as a lawyer, and he wasn't making too much money either.

Imogene Dick, Monticello

I was born in 1928 and raised in the Big Sinking Community here in Wayne County. I attended a two-room school there in Big Sinking. I finished all eight grades there at that school, then went to Wayne County High School and graduated in 1946. That high school was established in 1941. After high school was completed I went to Lindsey-Wilson College for two years, then later I went on to Eastern Kentucky University and graduated there. Some years later I went to Western Kentucky University and got my Head Start training. That was during one summer.

I taught in four one-room schools. My first year was at Gregory and I was paid $110 each month. After that I taught at Cedar Hill Schools for two years and my salary was $114 monthly, and I thought I was rich. My next year was at Rolly Creek where I taught one year, and then at Independence for two years.

All total, I taught school for forty-one years, and I'm now eighty years old.

Myrle Dunning, Marion

I graduated from Marion High School in 1948, then received a one-year scholarship to Western Kentucky State Teachers College. After the one year there, I did not have the money to go back to school the next year. I was contacted by the Crittenden County Board of Education and offered a job teaching at a school on the Ohio River known as Dam 50 School. I lived in Marion, and my dad and the men who operated Dam 50 helped to get me to and from school.

My first check for teaching there was fifty-three dollars monthly. My year there was the last year for the school. Dam 50 School closed and the families moved away.

After that year I became a secretary and later on an insurance agent here in Marion, Kentucky.

Nell S. Eaton, Glasgow

I attended a one-room school known as Clark's Corner, located in central Metcalfe County, during the years 1936–42. I then went to Edmonton High School and graduated in 1946.

I enrolled in Lindsey-Wilson College in Columbia, Kentucky, and was there in 1947–48. I then transferred in the fall, 1949, to Western Kentucky College, as it was known at that time, later becoming Western Kentucky University. I obtained my B.S. degree at Western in 1957, and my master's in 1959. I taught five years and did four years of college work during this time. I did summer terms and Saturday classes and all of the correspondence classes that I was allowed to take.

I taught one year at Walnut Hill one-room school, which had all eight grades. For eight years I taught at the consolidated school in Sulphur Well; served for five years as educational supervisor for Metcalfe County Schools; taught sixth, seventh, and eighth grade in Glasgow City Schools; served for nineteen years as Glasgow City Schools counselor; taught one and one-half years at Bowling Green Junior College in Glasgow; four years at Draughon's Junior College in Bowling Green; and taught English as second language to Japanese for seven and one-half years.

Norma Ramsey Eversole, Mt. Vernon

I was born in 1943 at Wildie, Rockcastle County. I attended Boiling Springs one-room school for the first five years of school, than a year and one-half at Wildie, also a one-room school, before completing elementary school at Mt. Vernon. I graduated second in my class from Mt. Vernon High School in 1961. After that I began substitute teaching at Cove in the fall, 1971, then went on to substitute in the other one-room schools the rest of that school year.

I taught in some of the schools for only a day or two at a time, while in others I sometimes stayed for two or three weeks. My pay was eleven dollars a day regardless of how far I had to drive or whether I had to keep the fire going or wash dishes. In monetary value I probably lost money, as I often supplemented the lunch menu from my own resources. However, the experience I received and the knowledge I gleaned from these often isolated communities were invaluable.

I enrolled in Eastern Kentucky University in 1972 and continued straight through summer, fall, and spring semesters until earning my degree in elementary education, December 1975.

Velois S. Fitts, Winchester

I was born August 10, 1921, in Mercer County, Kentucky. During my elementary years I attended Harrodsburg Elementary School, then graduated from Harrodsburg High School in 1939. I went to Bethel Women's College, a junior college located in Hopkinsville, then graduated from Pikeville College. After that I did my graduate work at Union College, Barbourville, with emphasis on special reading.

I chose to become a teacher because I always knew I wanted to be one. I truly loved the idea of becoming a teacher.

I grew up in Harrodsburg and taught schools there for several years before moving to Bell County, where I taught in a one-room school.

I taught in different schools a total of twenty years, then retired in 1958 or 1960.

My husband was a minister and teacher who taught at Clear Creek Baptist School, Bell County. We lived close to the Clear Creek School.

After retirement we moved to Winchester to be closer to our daughter, Deborah Condley, who is a librarian in Winchester. Our son, Dr. John Fitts, is a cardiologist in Bowling Green; another daughter is Suzanne Mantooth, a nurse and minister's wife in Morehead. Another son is Doug Fitts, a principal in Bell County.

Irma Gall, Barbourville

I was born in 1932 in northern Indiana, then came to Flat Creek, Clay County, Kentucky, in 1955 to work in a mission and teach after I graduated from Manchester College. I was a peace major, thus knew nothing at all about teaching school. At the same time I was living in Clay County, I taught in Leslie County for two years in a one-room school at Elifha Creek. It was part of Henry Ford's land over there, which is now the Red Bud Forestry Reserve. The school was in that reserve. After that I taught at Camp Creek up behind Windover, which was part of the Frontier Nursing Service.

All total, I taught ten years in one-room schools, three of which were in Knox County, and two in Leslie County.

Virginia Galloway, Merry Oaks

My father was born in eastern Kentucky but moved to Texas, and I was born in Wichita Falls, Texas, January 1914. We moved back here to Barren County when I was about three years old. I turned six in January, but back then kids didn't start school until they were six, and there were no preschools when I was growing up.

That fall I went to Carver, a one-room school near Railton here in Barren County. I went to school there during all my elementary years. After that I enrolled in a two-year country high school in Merry Oaks, located in western Barren County, when I was twelve years old.

After two years there, I enrolled in Western's College Heights High School in Bowling Green. I graduated from there in 1928. When I was eighteen years old, I started teaching at Carver School, a two-room school. I taught lower grades there for two or three years, then began teaching upper grades.

I taught at Red Cross one-room school for two years, then got married and lived in Bowling Green, but drove back to Red Cross every day, except for a day or so now and then when I stayed with my parents up here.

After Red Cross I taught at Cole's Bend one-room school, located near Barren River. All total, I taught in one-room schools for fifteen years. After that I taught in second grade for thirteen years at Red Cross once it had been consolidated. Subsequently, I went back to Western Kentucky University and earned my master's degree in library science. Thus I finished up my last five years in the library at the old Red Cross School.

I retired in 1975 after teaching for thirty-three and one-half years.

Many years ago, my dad taught some at Buck Creek one-room school. He was pretty well educated. He had a degree in law, but never practiced law. However, people came to see him from all over the neighborhood when they had a legal problem.

Grover C. Garland, London

I was born January 16, 1932, at Fogertown in Clay County. I attended a one-room school named Murray in 1937–38. After that I finished elementary school at a three-room school in Burning Springs, Kentucky. I then attended Bush High School, Laurel County, graduating in 1948. I then completed a two-year elementary teaching program at Sue Bennett College, located in London.

In the fall 1950 I began my teaching career at Sasser, a one-room school in Laurel County. To get there I drove a 1938 Chevrolet that belonged to my dad. The school was located on a gravel road. Next year I was transferred to Valley Grove, a one-room school closer to my home, but it was on a dirt road. To get there I had to walk about a mile or drive a farm tractor.

During my second year of teaching, the Korean "police action" was raging, and I was being drafted. In the middle of that school year I joined the U.S. Air Force and served for four years. That ended my one-room teaching days, but I would meet them again later.

At one time there were more than 101 two-room schools in Laurel County. By 1965, when I became a supervisor for the school system, that number was down to 14.

My pay during the year and one-half I taught in one-room schools was about $150 per month on a nine-month basis. However, it was enough that I was able to buy a two-year-old 1949 Chevrolet.

After my four years in the air force, I came home and attended the University of Kentucky. During that time, 1956–57, I taught one year at Clintonville, a consolidated elementary school in Bourbon County. I converted to secondary education, majoring in mathematics, with a second major in history and political science. Upon graduating from the University of Kentucky, I returned home to Laurel County and taught at Bush High School from 1957 to 1965. I taught math, but also served half-time as guidance counselor during the latter portion of that period. Also during that period I earned a master's degree at Eastern and attended several NDEA [National Defense Educational Act] institutes at various colleges.

In 1965 I was moved to the central office as a supervisor. That also happened to be the time of the "Great Society." Poverty was discovered in the Appalachian region and the ESEA [Elementary and Secondary Education Act] school programs were beginning. I then inherited the role of federal programs coordinator for the district. I wrote grants for Head Start programs, ESEA programs, and worked with NDEA projects from 1965 until 1978.

Patricia Gibson, Greenup

In 1950 I graduated from Prichard High School, Grayson, located in Carter County. That summer I began college at Morehead State Teachers' College (now Morehead State University). My sister-in-law and I commuted from Grayson to Morehead via Greyhound bus. At that time I-64 had not been constructed, so we traveled on U.S. 60. There were not many passing lanes, but there was a lot of truck traffic, and the trip was long and tedious.

It took me eleven years to complete my degree. I had married in 1950 and had four children during my eleven-year college experience. Another child came later. Besides one full year on campus, I attended weekend and/or night classes to achieve this. In 1961 I obtained my bachelor of arts degree, and had been teaching on a provisional elementary certificate during that time.

Garnet Gay Bailey Goble, Flat Gap

I was born in Johnson County, December 21, 1932. I personally attended one-room schools in Johnson County, which were Ramey's Branch, 1937–40, Joe's Creek, 1940–43, and McKenzie Branch, 1943–44. I then attended Flat Gap Elementary School and high school through the eleventh grade. I attended Meade Memorial High School during my twelfth year and graduated in May 1951. I enrolled at Berea College in September 1951. I married at the end of my sophomore year. Having sixty-four credit hours, I taught at Flat Gap Elementary, 1953–54.

My husband worked in Portsmouth, Ohio, so I moved there and did not teach for two years. In the meantime we had a lovely daughter in June 1955.

I began teaching at my first one-room school, the Head of Rush, in August 1955. I drove my car and then walked approximately one-half mile. The number of students in grades 1 through 8 ranged from fifteen to twenty. My first paycheck was in the amount of $125 each month, but I had to pay $40 for a babysitter.

I taught on an emergency teaching certificate for almost ten years. I began taking campus classes offered at Paintsville High School to renew the emergency certificate. I graduated from Morehead State College in 1962, then became a certified emergency education teacher, which gave me a substantial increase.

When the new government sponsored program under Title 11 became available to Johnson County schools, I was asked by the superintendent to accept a stipend of $300 to take classes at Morehead and move to a new consolidated school and teach the pilot program called the Educable Mentally Retarded. This was indeed an honor since I didn't have a certification at that time. The $300 was good for food and transportation. Tuition was also paid, as well as books and fees.

In 1968 Johnson County Schools built a new high school consolidating the three high schools, Meade Memorial, Flat Gap, and Oil Springs, along with the Van Lear Independent High School.

I retired in 1988 after teaching thirty years at Johnson County and Paintsville independent schools. I believe there is truth in the old adage "Children learn what they live."

Daphne H. Goodin, Barbourville

I was born in Knox County, February 14, 1934. I graduated from Union College with my first husband, who was killed in an automobile accident a few months later. I then remarried and was married for nineteen years, and we had a son in 1964. My husband died in 1980, and I have been a widow ever since.

I graduated from high school within three years by attending summer school two summers. I did not know much about Barbourville in my early years even though I lived only twelve miles away. . . . I got to thinking as I was going to summer school that there was something else in life other than washing on a washboard and being a wife and mother. I had no problem with the latter, as I wanted to be married and have kids. However, I wanted to do something else, so I crawled on a bus when I was sixteen, scared to death. I went to Cincinnati where I found a job the next day. I saved all my money to pay my college tuition in the fall, which was $220.

I finally got a job in the theater and worked there for five years while I was in college. I graduated from Union College in 1957 and started teaching at Knox Central High School. In 1964 I had to have a leave of absence because of being pregnant. I was called in September to substitute as a one-room school teacher because the teacher had been run off by students. I took the job. I went back to Union and earned my master's degree, then got my Rank 1 at Eastern Kentucky University. Then I went on and almost had enough hours to earn a doctor's degree, but I never did want to do a thesis.

I also have an administrative degree. I was the first women's physical education teacher and the first women's basketball coach in the whole district. I retired from teaching in January 1988 and started working for the Kentucky Education Association. I now work for teachers instead of students, but still do work that contributes to student achievement. I worked in other important positions for both state and local education organizations. My current real title is Uniserv director, as I serve six counties in southeastern Kentucky and eighty-five schools.

I have been working in education for fifty-one years. It has been a way of life for me. I taught for thirty years at Knox Central High School, coached girl's basketball for fifteen years, and taught in a one-room school for one year. I am past retirement age, but I still work and love it, as I feel I am still contributing something. All other wonderful activities aside, my year as a one-room school teacher stands out as the most memorable year of my life.

Maurine Everley Grant, Owensboro

I graduated from Rockport High School, Ohio County, May 1936, then attended Western Kentucky Teachers College, 1936–41. I received an elementary teacher's certificate in 1938, then taught for two years at Hickory Ridge one-room school and one year at Oakland one-room school. This was not a totally new experience, since I attended Ceralvo one-room school all of my elementary years.

In June 1941, I married my high school Casanova, Fred Grant, and received my bachelor of arts degree from what was then Western Kentucky Teacher's College in August 1941. I taught at Centertown High School one semester, then resigned to start a family. The next five years were spent caring for three beautiful children. . . .

In September 1947 I began teaching at Parkland Junior High School, Louisville. In 1962 I transferred to Valley High School at the time when double sessions were needed due to increased enrollments. My time schedule included a morning session, 7:00 a.m. to 1:00 p.m., and an evening session from 1:00 p.m. to 7:00 p.m. I experienced both sessions and can verify that it was not an ideal situation for teacher or students. In 1970 Jesse Stuart High School was constructed, so double sessions were no longer needed. I was assigned to teach science there, and did so until retirement in July 1976.

I have had a variety of experiences in my thirty-one years of teaching from one-room schools to high school, and also a variable salary. I am sure that it would be hard for teachers to believe the range of $64 a month, which was my beginning salary, to $14,725 per year, my highest salary.

Mayola Graves, Loretto

I went to St. Charles High School, then went to St. Catherine's College, Springfield, for two years. I started to college in 1932 at age eighteen. To be honest, I did not make all A's in my classes, but I took eighteen hours of courses all four semesters I was there. Thus, once I finished those two years I was qualified to be a schoolteacher.

I initially wanted to become a nurse, but in those days you had to go all the way to Louisville, so my parents objected to that. I knew I could go to St. Catherine's, so I went over there and boarded in a house while I was there. At that time my parents lived right here in Loretto, and this is where I was born at home, May 28, 1914. Loretto was settled by mostly Catholic persons back in early times.

My mother's maiden name was Emma Katherine Dant, and my daddy's name was Damian Hayden Buckler. They were both born in Marion County. My husband and I had seven children, one of which is deceased. Our children are college educated and have significant jobs. We have fourteen grandchildren and eight great grandchildren.

My teaching years were all taught in public schools, not Catholic. I was a very strict teacher. I taught with respect, and had very little trouble at any of the schools.

Duval Sidebottom Hay, Campbellsville

I was born July 26, 1923, in Green County. I attended Green County schools and taught in Green County schools. My first year of school was at Poplar Grove, back in 1929. I went three days, and the teacher had her son as a pupil and she beat him with a board, so I said, "I'm not going back any more because that teacher might kill you." So I set out that year. The next year we had a change of teachers, so my parents made me go to school.

I was going to be behind a year, but in 1937 they were offering a special eighth grade class in Greensburg, so I went there and took that special class. Upon graduation I went to Greensburg High School that fall and did my four high school years there, graduating in 1941.

I had my heart set on being a home demonstration agent, so I started to Campbellsville College during the fall 1941. I planned to go back to Campbellsville College beginning the next summer. However, Miss Nona Burris, who was the superintendent, sent word for me to come to town. School had been going on for five weeks, and I went into town to see what she wanted, and she said, "I need a teacher at Old Salem." I took the job, even though the two previous teachers were both run off by the schoolkids.

I went back to Campbellsville College when it became a senior college and got my B.S. degree there. By that time I was teaching at Greensburg Elementary School. After finishing at Campbellsville, I went to Western and got my Rank 1.

After my second child was born, my daughter started teaching at a one-room school at Gabe, and she called me and asked me to teach there my last year. I did, and taught fourteen children there. That was really a good school. Then I went to Summersville Elementary School and taught there for twenty-two years. I retired from teaching in 1981.

Pearl Helm, Russell Springs

I was born November 14, 1911, at Eli, Russell County. I attended a one-room school called Fonthill through the second grade; then my parents moved to Russell Springs where I finished grade and high school, graduating in 1930. After that I attended Lindsey-Wilson College for a whole year and actually received a two-year teacher's certificate in 1931.

Pearl McGowan was my maiden name. I married Howard Helm, who was later a Kentucky state representative.

I got a diploma at Lindsey-Wilson in May 1935, then taught at Wolf Creek one-room school. We had only six months of school that year because the county ran out of money. That was during Depression years. Years later Wolf Creek School was covered with water when Wolf Creek Dam and Lake Cumberland were built.

I taught at Wolf Creek for only one year, then taught at Beckham Ridge the next year. This school was near Russell Springs, so I walked to school from my home. I taught there for only one year, but didn't like it very well, thus thought about quitting as a teacher. So I skipped a year! However, that summer I substituted at Owenstown for one month and that was during the Russell County Fair. The teacher wanted to go to the Fair. Owenstown was destroyed by a tornado, I think in 1935.

Our family lived on Dr. Tarter's farm, and he knew I liked school. He loaned me money to pay my tuition at Lindsey-Wilson. After I started teaching that first year, I had to start paying him back, which also included interest. If I didn't pay on time, it was double interest!

I decided to start teaching once again, and my next teaching was for one year at a one-room school called Blair. After going to Lindsey-Wilson again, I taught at Grider

School for four years, then at French Valley School for one year. That gave me a total of eight years teaching in rural one-room schools.

I received a teaching certificate from Eastern Kentucky University in 1960, and continued teaching until I retired in 1972. All total, I taught at different schools for forty years.

Wanda Humble, Monticello

I actually didn't go to a one-room school. My first attendance was in a two-room school; then I graduated from Wayne County High School in 1950. Subsequently I attended Cumberland College, a two-year college, and graduated from there in 1952. I began teaching when I was eighteen years old, taught for ten years, then enrolled at Eastern Kentucky and received my B.S. degree there.

The first year I taught at a one-room school was Mt. Pisgah in 1952–53. Eighteen pupils were enrolled. My monthly check was $115, and I thought I was the richest human being that ever lived! Next year I moved to Missouri Hollow School, and taught there two years. I taught fifty-five students there, but Superintendent Ira Bell took all eighth-grade students to a three-room school due to the large number of students in Missouri Hollow.

After teaching in those two one-room schools, I took over teaching at Rocky Branch, an eight-room school, when Imogene Dick had to stop teaching for one-half year. For the rest of the year I taught at Rocky Branch, then for a total of sixteen years. After teaching there I began teaching at an elementary school and finished my career there, having taught for thirty-one years.

Virginia Janes, Edmonton

I used to walk to school when I was growing up in eastern Metcalfe County, near Highway 80. I went to school at Penick through the fifth grade, but after that I rode a bus and went to school in Edmonton through my sixth, seventh, and eighth grades. But when I later taught school at Penick, we had moved up close to my grandmother's, so I drove my daddy's car to school. He had an old '37 Ford, and it was really something!

I graduated from Edmonton High School in 1946, went to college at Western one year, and I taught that one year at Penick. I got married in December that first year I was teaching. Then I went to Lindsey-Wilson, a two-year college, and got my provisional certificate in 1949. After I started teaching I was going to school and teaching until five years before I retired. . . .

I took a lot of night and Saturday classes at Western, and also took some night classes at the University of Kentucky. I graduated from Western in 1959, then went on later and got my master's in 1969. I got my Rank 1 in 1977.

I taught for three years in one-room schools at Penick, Big Creek, and Angelly. I also taught for four years in Edmonton schools, which included first, second, and third grades. I taught the latter grade for two years, then the superintendent told me that a teacher was coming to Edmonton with her husband who was to be the new coach. The superintendent told me that this fellow's wife had never taught anything but third grade, so he planned to let her teach that grade. He asked me if I would teach the second grade, not the third grade. I said, "Well, she can have it."

After that I taught second grade, and taught it for twenty-seven years there in Edmonton. I retired from teaching in 1984.

Jimmie Jones, West Liberty

I was born August 29, 1941, in Lower Sand Lick, Morgan County. I have been married twice. My first wife was Brenda Gevedon, and we have two daughters, both of whom are social workers. My second wife is Theresa Williams Jones, a retired elementary school teacher.

I graduated from Morgan County High School in 1961, then attended Morehead State University, from which I received a bachelor's degree in 1961, a master's degree in 1975, and Rank 1 in 1978. I taught in a one-room school, 1965–66, then taught at Cannel City Elementary, 1966–89. While there I taught math, science, and social studies to seventh and eighth grades. At the end of that year all the elementary grades in Morgan County were sent to a consolidated middle school. I taught science to seventh-grade students at Morgan County Middle School, 1989–95, after which I retired from teaching.

Christine Thacker Justice, Mt. Sterling

I attended five different one-room schools in Pike County, then graduated from Feds Creek High School in 1946. Subsequently I attended Pikeville College from 1946 to 1948, then transferred to Eastern Kentucky State College, where I received my B.S. degree in 1952.

The community in which I grew up had only a few women who worked outside the home, and they were teachers. My mother often told me what I used to say as a child, with the words, "Mother, I'm going to be a teacher, then I'll buy you pretty clothes." At the age of five, I had already made up my mind about the future.

I taught school in Pike County for twenty-two years, then moved to Montgomery County in 1974. In the latter I was initially hired to be a special math teacher under the Title 1 program. I worked with fourth, fifth, and sixth graders who needed to improve their math skills. On the average, I had eight to ten per group. I witnessed progress, progress, progress, but that special program ended in 1976 after the local board of education decided to add more teachers to the special reading program rather than math.

I then began teaching language arts to sixth and seventh grades in the county's new middle school. There was a big difference in middle school students' attitude than what I had experienced. For example, I had always begun each morning with singing and the pledge to the flag. These middle school students weren't cooperative, and objected so badly that I had to give up my usual morning routine,

I retired in 1978, after a total of twenty-six teaching years.

Agnes Chandler Kenney, Walton

I was born January 16, 1900, in Rising Sun, Indiana. I began teaching in September 1918 at Verona School, located in Boone County, and I boarded with Mr. and Mrs. Craven, who lived near the school. After teaching at Verona, I taught at East Bend, Hume, Hamilton, Beaver Lick, and a new school at Verona. I taught for nine years and attended Eastern Kentucky State Teachers College. Some of my teaching also took place in two-room schools, which also included high schools situated in two-room structures. I stopped teaching in order to marry William Roy Kenney, June 1928. My husband was on the Boone County School Board in the early 1930s when they began consolidating the schools.

Georgia Lloyd, Barbourville
I was born in Pineville, Kentucky, 1932. My daddy had a restaurant, grocery store, and filling station in Pineville, but we moved to Barbourville when floodwaters got over the top of the building. Daddy just had everything shoveled out, sold everything, and moved to Barbourville.

As a little girl I attended city schools. At that time I didn't know there was such thing as one-room schools. I had not intended to become a teacher, even when I started to college. I graduated from Barbourville High School in 1949, then went to Union College and enrolled in the business department because I wanted to be a secretary and bookkeeper. When I married my husband, he had two years of college at the time, and they desperately needed teachers in Knox County. The superintendent asked him if he would like to teach at a school, and my husband said, "Well, I don't know anything about teaching."

The superintendent said, "Well, we need somebody since we don't have enough teachers." So my husband took the job.

I began teaching in 1951, taught in three one-room schools, in a two-room school, then taught in an elementary school during the rest of my career. I retired after forty-one years of teaching, and after that my daughter and I ran a gift and antique shop. We both enjoyed it, but it wasn't teaching. So I put an application in for substituting, and I substituted one hundred days each year for the next five years.

My husband said, "We won't be able to travel and do anything since you won't give up teaching." So I finally gave it up, but wasn't happy and still miss teaching. There is something about it that says it is what I was meant to do.

Across the years I taught three and one-half years in one-room schools; five years in a two-room school; five years in a four-room school; eight years in Barbourville City School (fourth grade); one year at Artemus Junior High School; eighteen years in Pineville City School (fourth grade); taught a summer term at Union College, 1987; then taught another summer term at Union College, 1988.

Pauline Keene Looney, Pikeville
I was born in 1931, and began my education in a one-room school named Miller's Creek, as did my two children. I graduated from Feds Creek High School in Pike County, then attended Pikeville Junior College (now Pikeville College) when it offered extension courses at Pikeville High School. That was in 1950; then I dropped out in 1951, but graduated in 1960 with a B.S. degree in elementary education.

I began substitute teaching in 1950, then married Harlow Looney in 1952, who died June 8, 2008. We parented a son, Stephen P. Looney, and a daughter, Sharon Looney McFeeley, and have four grandchildren, including one set of twins. Stephen is now vice president of a coal and mineral company, and is also a civil engineer. Sharon earned a degree in nuclear medicine, then worked first at Highlands Medical Center, Prestonsburg, then transferred from there to the Veterans Administration Hospital in Huntington, West Virginia.

Loella Lowery, Providence
I was born in Caldwell County in 1921. I graduated from Dawson Springs High School, then attended Western Kentucky Teachers College, 1939–41. I later returned to Western to get my B.S. degree in 1959.

My teaching career began in 1941 in Caldwell County at Hickory Ridge, a one-room school. It was a white building with long windows and a porch across the front. A bench sat on that porch. The school sat on a hill with houses down the hill from it. The schoolyard was rocky and had very little grass. The yard was never mowed while I was teaching there. It is not possible now to reach the site of the school by vehicle.

I taught for forty-one years, then retired June 30, 1983.

Betty Jo Arnett Lykins, Salyersville

I was born August 7, 1936, in Magoffin County. I attended Rudd School all of my elementary years, then graduated from Salyersville High School in 1954. I attended Lees Junior College, Prestonsburg Community College, Morehead State University, and the University of Kentucky. I received an A.B. degree, M.A. degree, and Rank 1 at Morehead State University, then did postgraduate work at the University of Kentucky.

I taught two years in one-room schools in Magoffin County, then taught an additional thirty years in the Magoffin Public School System. The system was consolidated in 1964. Subjects I taught at various locations included early childhood education, and language arts and social studies in a middle school. During the last four years of my career, I worked in the central office as coordinator of writing and gifted education.

I retired from the public school system in 1997, then after 2000 I taught in a private school for Muslim children. We used the one-room concept, teaching all subjects in a self-contained classroom. We taught Kentucky Core Curriculum.

That was a positive experience, as I had come full circle. I stopped teaching in 2007, but am presently a social activist, promoting regional literature and better environmental practices. My hobbies are reading, writing, sewing, and loving my grandchildren.

I have been married to J. L. Lykins since 1955, and we have three sons and three daughters, eight grandchildren, and two great-grandchildren.

Stella K. Marcum, Pikeville

I was born May 23, 1943, at Fishtrap, Pike County, the daughter of Nathaniel and Jettie Kendrick. There were nine children in my family, five girls and four boys. I was next to the oldest, and the only one to receive a college degree. I attended Feds Creek High School and graduated in 1961.

I stayed out of school one semester; then I enrolled at Pikeville College in January 1962. One year later I married Allen Marcum, also a Pikeville college graduate. He taught school in New Lebanon, Ohio, for one year, then after our marriage he returned to Pikeville and worked as an insurance adjustor for forty-five years. Allen and I have one son, George Allen Marcum, who is also a Pikeville College graduate, and works as a supervisor with Chesapeake Energy (a natural gas company) near Prestonsburg, Floyd County.

I began teaching in a one-room school at Lower Elk of Knox Creek, Kentucky, at the age of twenty-one, with an emergency teaching certificate. I returned to Pikeville College during the 1965–66 school year to finish my senior year and required student teaching. The latter was performed at Betsy Lane High School, Floyd County. I received my degree in business education at Pikeville College on June 5, 1966.

I began teaching math in the seventh and eighth grades at Elkhorn City School, located in that city, during the fall, 1966. I taught there for nine years, then transferred to Millard High School in Pike County, where I taught math and algebra in the same school grades for seventeen years.

I retired in 1992 at the age of forty-nine, after twenty-seven years of teaching in Pike County schools.

Betty Holmes McClendon, Nancy

I was born March 28, 1928. I attended Somerset High School, from which I graduated in 1944. In 1947 I attended a six weeks' workshop in Somerset. There were experienced teachers who taught basic subjects that exposed our group to as much review as possible in the length of time we were together. This prepared me for all duties I acquired to teach my first year of first- to eighth-grade students.

In 1948 I attended Lindsey-Wilson Junior College during the spring quarter, then began teaching at McClendon School, one-room. Interspersed with attending spring terms, summer terms, and some off-campus classes, I received my provisional elementary teaching certificate. Then I started attending Eastern Kentucky College and graduated from there in 1960. I never attended a full semester of college at one time. Local night classes, Saturday classes at Eastern, along with summer terms there, gave me hours I needed to graduate with a B.S. degree.

I taught special reading at Nancy Elementary School for fourteen years. When I retired in 1979, after thirty-one and one-half years of teaching in various schools, I was presented a silver tray by one of my former McClendon School students, Darrell Beshears, county judge at the time.

I married Arnold McClendon. Our daughter, Rebecca Ann, was born in June 1955. She began school at age five. In 1962 she was diagnosed with leukemia and died in September 1963.

The only family member that also taught in a one-room school was my sister Louise, but cousins on both sides of my family have pursued teaching careers.

Pat McDonald, Barbourville

I was born January 8, 1938, and grew up in the Little Brush Creek community here in Knox County. I attended a one-room school for four years, then enrolled in Barbourville Elementary School due to our moving into Barbourville after my dad came home after World War II. He enrolled at Union College, so I went to the city school for two years. After that we went back to Brush Creek, and I attended Artemus Elementary School during the seventh and eighth grades.

I attended Knox Central High School and graduated in 1956. I wanted to be a veterinarian, then wanted to be a doctor, but couldn't get the right courses at Knox Central. I attended the University of Florida for one semester, but got homesick and came back here to enroll in Union College. I enrolled there in 1957 and graduated in 1960. I majored in history, political science, and physical education.

I began teaching in a one-room school called Davis Bend. I taught one year there, but then they asked me to teach history and social studies at Knox Central. After that I began traveling around. I went to Gray Elementary and taught there, as I was the only person that had an elementary physical education degree in the county. I stayed there for four years and started basketball and football, also a track team.

The county built a new school on north Highway 11 at Girdler, and I taught there five years; then they built the G. R. Hampton School and I was transferred there to start athletic teams and teach physical education. I stayed there for four years, but in the meantime I got my master's degree at Union College in 1966. After that I attended Eastern Kentucky University and got a Rank 1 certification.

In 1974 I got a job in the central office in Knox County as director of pupil personnel. I worked in that position for twenty-one years, and had already taught for fourteen years—thus I worked in the school business for thirty-five years, then retired in 1995.

I used my first paycheck to buy my future wife an engagement ring. We got married when she was seventeen years old, in 1960. I was teaching in the one-room when we got married. She was a sophomore at Union College, so she went on to become a teacher also.

Grace W. McGaughey, Lexington

I was born January 28, 1920. I attended Deckard one-room school, then graduated from Rineyville High School in 1939. However, before that my family moved to Harrison County, Indiana, near Palmyra, when I was four years old. I was inspired by a teenage girl there to go to college and become a teacher. At an early age I made up my mind to become a teacher; then as a high school student I decided to go to Western Kentucky State College. I received an early teaching certificate, then renewed my certificate by taking a Kentucky history course at the University of Kentucky and an American history course at Western. I then taught for one-half year at Sulphur Elementary School, Henry County; then, after taking six hours at Georgetown College, I taught at Eminence, Henry County, for three years. Soon thereafter my husband, William, was transferred to Hazard, so I taught in Perry County at Walkertown Elementary School.

After three years there my husband was transferred to Bardstown, and while there I attended Nazareth College and taught remedial reading and physical education in first and second grades. After we then moved to Lexington, I attended the University of Kentucky and became a qualified librarian. I then served as a day-shift librarian at Lafayette Junior High School, and also at a new junior high school, Jesse Clark. In 1967 I received my M.S.L.S. degree in library science.

When my husband was transferred to Indianapolis, I taught one year there in an elementary school, and served as librarian two and one-half years in two high schools. After that my husband was transferred to Washington, D.C., as an RC and D [Rural Conservation and Development] specialist. I then applied for a public library position in Manassas, Virginia, but it had been filled. They called me from the Manassas Library about a school library at Elizabeth Vaughan that had an opening due to the librarian's resignation after she married. I got that job in January 1973. I stayed there six and one-half years until William retired in 1978.

We moved back to Lexington, where I served in 1979 as teacher and librarian. In 1980 I taught a split class of fifth and sixth grades at Johnson Elementary School, then served as librarian at Russell Cave Elementary School, Fayette County, for four years.

I retired in 1984 after serving as teacher/librarian in thirteen schools in Kentucky, Indiana, and Virginia.

Michael M. Meredith, Bee Spring

I graduated from Kyrock High School in 1955, then enrolled at Western Kentucky University in 1955, and eventually finished with B.A., master's, and counseling degrees in 1982.

My mother was a teacher who graduated from Western in 1928. She taught at Jock School and rode a horse from Bee Spring to Jock in order to get there.

The first one-room school at which I taught was Bee Spring Elementary. I drove a 1950 Ford in order to get there, and my teaching salary was $200 per month. When I began teaching I had twenty-nine students and was teaching on an emergency certificate. After this I went back to Kyrock, where I initially taught a combination of fourth- and fifth-grade students.

After I received my first degree from Western Kentucky University, I went to Lincoln Elementary as head teacher and coach. We had 150 students and I stayed there for seven years.

I attended Indiana University in order to obtain more hours on my degree. After that, and after working for a period of time for Ralph Myers Construction Company, I decided to go back to teaching. I received an offer to teach for seven months in another one-room school, located in Sadler, Grayson County. The last two months that year were spent teaching at Chalybeate Elementary, Edmonson County.

After teaching at Bee Spring, Kyrock Elementary, Lincoln Elementary, and Sadler Elementary, I returned to Kyrock Elementary and remained there until I retired in 1992.

Noble H. Midkiff, Whitesville

I graduated from Fordsville High School in 1937. On July 20, 1939, at age nineteen, I began teaching my first school in a rural area. The next month, August 30, I turned twenty years old. I acquired a teaching certificate from Western Kentucky College in 1939, a B.S. degree in 1949, my master's degree in 1961, then got my Rank 1 in 1974.

I decided to become a teacher because I love children, and it is a very calling vocation. Teaching was a great asset to me across the years.

In late 1941 I went to Sorgho Elementary, located in Daviess County, and taught there until I was drafted into the army in 1942. While I was in the army, my wife and I went thirty-three months and ten days without laying eyes on each other. I got my first wound February 1, 1943, in North Africa. I got my second combat wound July 12, 1944, in Italy, and I got my right ankle all tore up April 17, 1945, north of Florence, Italy. I was in the army hospital about five days, and I almost didn't make it. The United States did its part, and I'm so thankful.

I taught vocational agriculture for sixteen and one-half years at Home High School, Fordsville, beginning in January 1949. After that I served as principal at the Fordsville Elementary and High School, 1962–70. Subsequently the Ohio County superintendent assigned me to the central office to do the federal program for all Ohio County schools, 1970–75. I decided to retire when I was only fifty-six years old.

During all that time I farmed, raised tobacco, had cattle, and sold feeder pigs.

My wife, Jewel, who was my best friend and partner for sixty-two and one-half years, passed away on May 8, 2004. We have three children, seven grandchildren, and five great-granddaughters.

At eighty-nine years old, I'm so thankful I can still do things that I enjoy.

J. Robert Miller, Rock Bridge

Named John Robert Miller but known as J. Robert Miller, I was born in Monroe County, June 5, 1920, to Harlan Ross Miller and Ina (Chapman) Miller, a one-room school teacher at Hickory Ridge, Monroe County. I graduated from Gamaliel High School in 1939, briefly attended Western Kentucky Teachers College, then taught in 1941 at Oak Hill one-room school and for three months at Hamilton one-room school in 1942 prior to being drafted into military service, in which I served for three and one-half years. Subsequently I graduated from Western in 1948 with a B.S. degree in agriculture. I then taught at Tompkinsville High School, 1948–67, during which time I earned a master's degree in agriculture in 1955 at the University of Kentucky. In November 1967 I was elected as Kentucky commissioner of agriculture and served through 1971. No other Monroe Countian has been elected to a statewide position. I served as a life insurance salesman for several years while also engaged in farming.

I married Naomi Bowman and we became parents of Roberta (Miller) Eldred; Johnny, who worked in the Monroe County Health Department; Rhoda Beth (Miller) Huffman; and Joseph Jesse, who worked for the federal government in the Department of Defense.

I have been a member of numerous state boards and commissions, as well as local organizations, across the years, including the Monroe County Historical and Genealogical Society.

Hale Murphy, Eddyville

I was born September 25, 1925, in Eddyville, Kentucky. I attended Moulton one-room school, located in the Confederate community, then Eddyville High School, from which I graduated in 1944. I then attended Western Kentucky University for one quarter of time. I was offered a teaching job at Bruce School on the basis of an emergency certificate. That was during World War II, and I was classified 4-F, and was glad to get a job. I attended Western Kentucky again in 1945, but without a degree.

During the war Lyon County had several emergency teachers. I was still at home and drove my dad's pickup truck to Bruce School every day. The pay was seventy-five dollars a month. School was held for seven months, July through January. I played games with the students, most of which were ball games. We sometimes walked to Dewey School to play ball against them.

I married Dollie Hester February 10, 1945. We have three children and four grandchildren. In regards to my ancestors and other relatives, including my wife, many were teachers. My great-grandfather, Sam Hooks, taught in Trigg County. My great-grandmother Malinda Cunningham married Sam, who was her teacher, and they later moved to Lyon County. Their daughter, Minnie, married Seldon Murphy, and they became parents of my aunt Ruth, who taught at Moulton, a school that was founded in 1840 and remained active until it was closed in 1951–52.

My family and I left Lyon County in 1946 and lived in Louisville for forty-plus years. I worked for State Farm Insurance in various capacities, but never taught schools after 1944–45. I retired in 1987. My wife, Dollie, obtained her college degree from the University of Louisville and taught in Jefferson County schools, 1963–82. We came home to Eddyville in 1987, and have lived here every since.

Alma New, Monticello

I was born in 1921. I went to a one-room school all eight grades, and to the same teacher, Olivia Higgenbotham. After that I attended three high schools here in Wayne County. I boarded in a home during my first high school year at Parmelyville because it was too far from home and I didn't have any way of getting to school. From there I attended Rocky Branch High School, and went to school there until the new Wayne County High School was built in Monticello, and it was from the latter that I graduated in 1942.

I went to college at Lindsey-Wilson for two years, then to Western Kentucky University for two years and obtained a B.S. degree. I taught at Gregory one-room school for two years, beginning in 1943, and I think my first check was sixty-seven dollars. After my second year there Dad and Mom sold our farm and moved to Indianapolis. I was in college there at the time, so I wrote a letter to Superintendent Ira Bell asking him if he had a school where I could teach, since I'd like to return home to Wayne County to teach.

I got a letter back from him telling me yes, that I could have Rolly Creek School, and I could board with my grandmother who lived about one mile from the school. So I taught there.

Next year I got married and lived there and taught at Gregory School again. Then the next year I taught at Big Sinking School, which was farther on up from where I lived.

All total, I taught thirty years, five of which were in one-room schools. Their names were Gregory, Rolly Creek, and Big Sinking.

William H. Nicholls Jr., The Villages, Fla.

I was born in Taylorsville, Spencer County, September 30, 1930. I graduated from Taylorsville High School in 1948 as one of thirty-five students, then began teaching at Fairview one-room school located in the eastern part of the county. I was seventeen years old at that time, but turned eighteen that fall. I attended Georgetown College summer terms in 1948, and taught at Fairview during regular school months.

My teaching career was cut short when I returned full-time to Georgetown in 1949 to prepare for entrance to the U.S. Naval Academy, an offer I could not refuse. I graduated from Annapolis in 1954 with a B.S. degree and was commissioned in the U.S. Navy. I graduated from the Rensselaer Polytechnic Institute, Troy, New York, in 1957, with a B.C.E.

I retired from the Navy Civil Engineer Corps in 1974, then served as a civil engineer at Ronald Reagan Washington National and Washington Dulles International airports, 1974–95. Upon retirement from that position, I was a self-employed civil engineer, 1995–2003, in Virginia Beach, Virginia.

Upon retirement I moved to The Villages, Florida, which is my current place of residence.

I married Betty Pennington of Annapolis on July 2, 1954. We became the parents of two children, and now have four grandchildren.

Betty Jane (Miller) Pence, Franklin, Tenn.

I was born in Rock Bridge, Monroe County, in the house where I grew up and lived until I married in 1951. As to the morning when I was born, my mother always said she did the wash that morning, then she realized I was on my way. So my dad sent for a doctor, but I think I was born before he arrived.

My mother was Ina Floe Chapman, and she married my father, Harlan Ross Miller. I have teacher heritage in my family, as my grandfather Miller was a teacher, and my mother was a teacher. One of my brothers, Robert, was also a teacher.

I became a teacher quite by accident, because I was in college at the time when Superintendent Zeke Harlan came out to my home one summer. He had been my teacher in high school and knew I was in college. It was time for school to start, as rural schools always started in July. Actually, I was planning to go back to college, as I had only completed two years. Mr. Harlan said to me, "I have a one-room school I don't have a teacher for. It's close to you, and I really need for you to teach."

I guess the idea of making the first money I ever did appealed to me, so I gave in and went to Bowman School and taught. Had I not attended a one-room school myself, I would have had no idea as what to do. I taught one year there in 1949, then taught at Union Hill for one year.

After I taught at Bowman School and Union Hill one-room school, I went back to Western and finished my third year; then I got married. I never finished college, but I worked in school offices in later years, and worked in Florida in a reading tutoring program. I have also done that as a volunteer in Williamson County, Tennessee.

After I married in 1951, I followed my husband, Jim, all over the world, because he was career military. I lost out on details as to which one-room schools were closed, but later on I was really sad when I saw that one-room Merryville School there in Rock Bridge had been torn down.

Helen Raby, Elizabethtown

I was born in 1915 in Springfield, Tennessee, and lived there for four years; then we moved to Adairville, Logan County. Adairville is where I went to school all twelve years. After I graduated in 1934, I was interested in becoming a teacher, primarily because I had three great teachers and wanted to imitate them if I could. I started to Western Kentucky College in September 1935 and went one year.

At that time it was awfully hard to get a teaching job at a school. My uncle gave me a teaching job, and I was wanting to make enough money. I took the job in 1936 and taught there for two years. I got married and had two children, Rodney and Janet, thus didn't teach for awhile until my children got old enough to go to school. I started again, then received a degree from Western in the 1950s, the same year I turned forty.

My son, Rodney, was Kentucky State Fire Marshall for thirty-three years. My daughter, Janet, and her daughter, Kari Harwell, are speech therapists in Adairville. What they do is work on children that can't talk. What they do is wonderful.

I taught school for thirty-one years, and after that, my good friend who was principal at Russellville asked me if I would do some substitute teaching. I told him I would, then substituted for eighteen years. That was an average of about three days a week. When he needed more than one substitute, he was partial to me.

All total, I had forty-nine years of teaching, most of which were in Russellville.

Lucille Hoover Ringley, Monticello

I was born December 12, 1928, in Powersburg, Wayne County. I attended Jennings Hollow and Windy one-room schools, then attended Wayne County High School, from which I graduated in 1946. After high school I was permitted to enter Cumberland Junior College a few days after the second semester began, with the understanding that I would make up all the work I had missed in each class. I did this in January 1948 and January 1949, then graduated from Cumberland Junior College in May 1949.

I was able to finish my college work as long as the school year was seven months

Biographies of Storytellers

long by entering the college during spring term, and sometimes working on a summer term. I kept this pace up for six years, at which time the Lord brought a wonderful, handsome young navy man into my life, and we were married August 27, 1952. I traveled with him and was employed by the navy for the next three years. Then we returned to Kentucky and had three wonderful children. I did not teach any full-time jobs until I finished correspondence courses, and by commuting to Williamsburg and Richmond to earn my B.S. degree. I later earned my master's degree and Rank 1.

At that time I was hired at Monticello Independent Schools, from which I retired due to health problems in 1990. I finished thirty-two years of service, including my years teaching in four different one-room schools in Wayne County. These schools were Jennings Hollow, Denney Hollow, Waite, and Windy.

My mother, Ora Bertram Hoover, also helped in one-room schools as a teacher's aide.

Gladys H. Roy, Columbia

I was born November 27, 1923, in Wayne County. I attended Hancock School, a one-room school located in the hills of Wayne County. I walked to and from school, as the roads were rough and no one in that area had transportation. I attended Windy High School for two years, which was a country high school. I had to walk a long way to catch a bus. After two years there, our county high schools, three in number, were consolidated into Wayne County High School, located just outside Monticello. I rode a bus about thirteen miles each way, but had to walk two miles to get to the bus stop. I graduated from high school in 1943.

Upon graduation I attended a business college in Nashville, Tennessee, 1943–44, then taught for awhile. Later on I attended Lindsey-Wilson College in Columbia, that operated on a quarter-term system. I managed to keep getting college credits toward my degree by attending summer school and Saturday classes. Upon completion of my two years at Lindsey-Wilson, I taught for three years. I took correspondence courses and later enrolled at Western Kentucky Teachers College and received a B.S. degree. Then in 1953 I received a master's degree equivalent.

I retired in 1981 after teaching eleven years in one-room schools and twenty years in elementary and high schools, but I also substituted until 2008, when I was eighty-five years old.

Zona Royse, Columbia

I was born December 9, 1934, in Russell County. My father was a farmer, so we moved around in that part of the county in which we lived. We lived in Horseshoe Hollow when I was very young, but moved away from that area when I was four or five years due to the coming of Wolf Creek Dam and Lake Cumberland.

Mother's name was Bessie Dixon Bradshaw, and my daddy was Ive Lee Bradshaw. Both were natives of Russell County. Mother was a teacher, so I was actually home-schooled during the first grade. She got her books and taught me first grade at home because she couldn't lift my brother, due to the TB that she had. My older brothers and sisters went on to school while she taught me at home.

I started to Blair School during the second grade. I went to that school until I was ready to go into sixth grade. I did go to school that year for six weeks, but since my brother played basketball at Jamestown, my mother sent me there to school. That year we had our first school bus, and we had to walk a mile and one-half to catch it, and since it was privately owned we had to pay $1.27 per week to ride it.

Since I had already gone to the sixth grade for a few weeks, I skipped the rest of it that year and went on into the seventh grade. I did seventh and eighth grade at Jamestown Elementary School. When I started as a freshman at Russell Springs High School, the county began to provide free bus service. My brother and I were in the same grade during our senior year in high school. He was older than I, but we graduated together since I had skipped sixth grade.

I started college at Lindsey-Wilson in 1952, and graduated from there in 1954 with an associate arts degree in elementary education. After that I got married and got a teaching job in Adair County, where I taught for thirty-eight years.

After I taught for awhile they told me I had to get a B.S. degree, so then I enrolled at Western in Bowling Green. I got some of my credits from Western, and then Campbellsville College had elevated to a four-year college, so I transferred to Campbellsville, located fairly close to us. I got my B.D. degree there, but went back to Western and received my master's degree and Rank 1 in the 1970s.

Bernice Shartzer, Caneyville

I was born at home in Caneyville, June 6, 1912. At that time my parents were renting a house in Caneyville. My father was Oscar Smith, and my mother was Myrtle Poole Smith.

At age six I went my first day of school at Stinson School, a one-room building that is still standing. I went there to school through the eighth grade. Later on I taught my first year there in 1930. I married Arnold Shartzer in 1934, and we moved to our farm in 1936. The farm included a hill called Cat Route because it was a hill that was so steep a cat was all that could walk across the hill.

In order to go to high school, I had to take two diploma examinations. We had to do that in order for the county to pay our tuition to the independent high school. Thus I rode a train to Leitchfield, where I took the diploma examinations. That got me started, so I went on to high school at Caneyville and graduated from there in 1930. At that time Grayson County didn't have a high school. Caneyville was an independent school district, as were Leitchfield and Clarkson.

I went to college at Odgen College in Bowling Green and received a two-year certificate on sixteen hours of credit. After that I went back to get my lifetime teaching certificate. I taught in the fall, and went back to school in the spring.

When my two daughters were preteens, I went to Western and took Saturday classes and evening classes and got my bachelor's degree.

I taught at several one-room schools, which included Walnut Grove, where the old building is still standing. I began teaching in one-room schools in 1930 and did so until 1952. The one-room schools at which I taught were Stinson, Ned Springs, Bates, Freedom, Walnut Grove, Millwood, Spring Lick, and Lewis. I also taught at Wilson School in Butler County. My last one-room teaching took place in 1952–53 at Stinson. All total, I taught sixteen years in one-room schools, and two years in two-room schools, which were Spring Lick and Millwood.

I started teaching in Caneyville in 1954, when it was consolidated. One-room schools were being closed gradually in the 1950s. I retired from teaching in 1973, but did some substitute teaching until I fell and broke my hip in 1985.

Mattie Jo Smith, Benton

I was born in 1918 in Marshall County near Benton, the county seat. My mother graduated from Benton High School in 1917. Her two aunts became teachers and taught in several of the county's schools. One taught seventh grade in the Butler Independent District in 1948, then later taught one year at Breezeel School.

My family lived in the Benton Independent District, which for some years had the only high school in Marshall County. I graduated from Benton High School in 1936 and entered Murray State Teachers College in the fall 1936. I earned a teaching certificate in two years and began teaching at Breezeel one-room school for a salary of sixty-four dollars per month.

The seven-month school term began in July and ended in January. I was able to enroll during the spring semester at Murray in February 1939. My father, who had very little formal education, insisted I become a teacher. Any girl who graduated from high school and could manage tuition costs at Murray became a teacher. Those were Depression years. I did live in one of the student rooming houses in Murray. From home, I took lots of food to eat.

Each school in Marshall County had a trustee who hired the teachers. Most beginning teachers were hired for two years, so I taught two years at Breezeel. The first year there, there were fifty students enrolled. The eighth grade had nine boys and three girls, and they were all bigger than I.

After World War II I taught a third year at Breezeel. My four-year-old daughter went with me. Murray College had become Murray State University, and I enrolled there again in 1952. I was hired by the Benton Independent Schools as a junior high math and English teacher. I finished my B.S. degree in education in 1957 and taught for twenty-six years. I retired in 1980 with a total of thirty years service.

Hilda Snider, Taylorsville

I was born December 15, 1927, in Spencer County to Rufus and Ruby Miller Greer. I am their middle child; I have a sister and brother. At the age of five I entered a one-room school in Nelson County and was there for three years, then completed elementary years in a two-room school. I attended Mount Eden High School one year, then graduated from Taylorsville High School in 1945.

After graduation I worked in the Taylorsville Post Office, then married Orval Snyder of Mount Eden in December 1945. Soon thereafter I began teaching in a one-room school on Salt River. During that first year of teaching I took two college courses by correspondence; then the following summer I enrolled in Spalding College, Louisville, to begin my work on a degree in elementary education. I received my B.S. degree in May 1959.

Our son, John Mark Snider Sr., was born in 1958. After taking a leave of absence for one year, I returned to the classroom. Not long thereafter I began working on my master's degree, thus took classes at Spalding University, Eastern Kentucky University, and some extension classes. I received my master's in 1971 and Rank 1 in 1975—principalship and administration, with emphasis on supervision.

Across the years I taught history, typing, and bookkeeping at Taylorsville High School for one year, then taught eighth grade the next year. The following year I taught fifth grade in Bullitt County, and after that I was hired in the Jefferson County school system, where I stayed until retirement. While in Jefferson County I served as instructional supervisor and as a reading resource teacher. I taught first, third, and fifth grades at Bates Elementary School on Bardstown Road.

I have served in positions at Taylorsville's First Baptist Church, and as a member of D.A.R., Spencer County Historical Society, Kentucky Retired Teachers Association, and other clubs of interest. I am also involved in many community activities.

My sister is also a retired teacher, having worked twenty-eight years in Bullitt County as a teacher and supervisor. My dad had two cousins who taught almost fifty years in Granite City, Illinois.

Laura Agnes Townsley Stacy, Barbourville

I was born September 8, 1929, in Hammond, Kentucky, located in Knox County. Later that community came to be knows as Barnyard, and it had a post office. I am one of fifteen children, six boys and nine girls, born to Julia Belle Smith and John Anderson Townsley. Three of the boys died as infants.

The first half-year I went to school was in a log cabin called Hinkle Branch School. I went to a two-room school the rest of that year, and it was called Jackson School. My first year of high school was at Flat Lick, where they had a first-year high school. I then attended Knox Central High School and graduated in 1948.

The day I started to high school, when I hadn't much more than ever left Stinking Creek at that time, except my first trip to Barbourville was in a wagon drawn by mules. I enrolled at Union College during the summer 1947, and took two courses for a total of seven hours. That was the end of my college until later, after I had married and had two children. I didn't go back to college until our kids were in school. I was a stay-at-home mom.

Our income wasn't too good because my husband was a laborer and didn't make very much money. I saw right away that I was going to have to help out with our finances, so I started back to college and got placed in these one-room schools until I got my degree in 1966. When I received my degree I was sent to four-room New Bethel School where I taught third and fourth grades, and that was a blessing.

I decided to become a schoolteacher after I had applied for jobs in different places and didn't get a job. During my first years in one-room schools I taught with an emergency certificate. My first one was at Sprule School, located on Bull Creek, where I began in November. The reason I was employed to teach there was because they had run the teacher off. That school had all eight grades.

I received my master's degree in 1970, with emphasis in reading. I taught special reading for two years at Girdler Elementary School. In 1978 I received my Rank 1 degree in library science. From that point on I served as librarian at Girdler Elementary until my retirement in 1991. Since then I have done substitute teaching in Knox County.

Bernadine Shirley Sullivan, Campbellsville

I was born October 22, 1925, in Green County, but my parents moved to Metcalfe County two years later, where I spent the next twenty years of my life. We lived at the point where Adair, Green, and Metcalfe counties come together. I went to a one-room school in Adair County my first year, called Keltner School.

The next year I either went to New Era or Stony Point, which were about the same distance from our house. I graduated from New Era in 1939 and started to Greensburg High School that fall, graduating in 1944. At that time I felt like I wanted to become a secretary.

My sister and her husband were living in Indianapolis, and he was in the army. I went up there and spent a week, bored stiff, and didn't find a job. I decided to become a schoolteacher, so I came home. Somehow or another, Dad found enough money to pay my tuition at Lindsey-Wilson College that summer, which was 1944. At that time the United States was at war, and schoolteachers weren't to be found. Thus schools could just take anybody as a schoolteacher.

I went to school for six weeks at Lindsey-Wilson, then started looking for a place to teach. Well, they found a school for me in Hardin County out in the boonies, or way back in the hills. My dad took me back there, and I found a couple who were fifty-three and fifty-four years old when I went there. I lived with them during that school year. The school was called Osborne. During the war I had students in the first grade who were nine years old! They had not had school in that area for three years.

I finished the school year there, then came back home and attended Lindsey-Wilson College. My next school was at New Era, from which I had graduated. I was staying with my parents.

The next year, 1946, I taught at Stony Point, which was a school I had gone to as a child. The next year I received a provisional certificate from Lindsey-Wilson, then taught at Liletown School in Green County. I was dating my husband-to-be at that time. He had taken me home from Lindsey-Wilson one night after a date, and I had gotten this letter stating I had been hired to teach at Liletown. So I yelled out the window to him and said, "I've got a Liletown School in Green County."

Liletown is where he had gone to school, so he said, "Oh, they'll kill you; they'll kill you. That school is really rough."

Anyway, I went there in 1947, the same year we had married and moved into that area. All total, I taught at Liletown, Buckner, and Lone Oak, and rotated between the three each year.

All that time I was going back to school during the summer, and I did some school-work by correspondence. I received my bachelor's degree in 1958; then my husband said, "Well, while you are into it, you might as well go ahead and get your master's degree." So I did, and got my master's degree at Western Kentucky University in 1960.

In 1960 I began teaching eighth grade in Greensburg Elementary School. Basically, I taught English, reading, spelling, and whatever. Later on I shifted to the sixth grade, and when I got to the point where I was about ready to retire, the superintendent wanted me to shift down, so he put me in the fifth grade. I didn't want to make that change, so I went to Superintendent Buddy Lowe and cited and pleaded, but it did no good. So I finished my last three years in the fifth grade.

I started teaching in 1944 and quit in 1988, after teaching for forty-four years, sixteen of which were one-room schools, from 1944 to 1960.

Back then, if a student wanted consolation, you could give them a hug, but now it's a little different.

Thomas "Rube" Tackett, Prestonsburg

After teaching at Goble Branch one-room school until it was closed in 1960, I returned to Morehead State College to finish my A.B. degree so that I could teach high school classes. Two years later I was hired at Prestonsburg High School to teach American history and civics. Three years later with a master's degree in principalship, I was hired as principal at Prestonsburg Elementary.

From 1965 to 1990 I worked with boys and girls as they learned and grew up. In 1990 we built a new middle school and I became principal. In 1992 I was demoted and spent the next three years teaching homebound students throughout Floyd County. During those three years I filed a lawsuit against the Floyd County Board of Education and won. The board of education paid me three years back pay, apologized, and was ordered to reinstate me as principal at the middle school. By this time site-based councils were hiring principals.

One night my doorbell rang. When I opened the door there were three teachers and two parents from Prestonsburg High School. I thought they were looking for a donation since I had won many thousands of dollars from the school board. They didn't want money; they wanted me to be their principal. I told them that for twenty-five years I had tied shoestrings, put on band-aids, and made sure every child caught their school bus home. I went on to say that during my two years at the middle school each young person was important, and their future was of great concern to their parents, teachers, and me. With a few questions, I determined that perhaps what Prestonsburg High School needed more than anything else was a leader to convince students of their worth and pride in themselves and their future. Thus, I accepted the job as Prestonsburg High School principal.

I stayed three years and worked with many wonderful students, teachers, and parents. I retired in 1998, but as I look back I realize that the twelve students at a one-room school on Goble Branch taught a "green behind the ears" nineteen-year-old to love teaching boys and girls.

Vera Virgin, Greenup

I was born August 16, 1915, in Lime Hollow, Greenup County, Kentucky, to parents Virgil Rezin Virgin and Della Bays Virgin. I was child number nine in a family of eleven brothers and sisters. We had no modern conveniences, no electricity, no bathrooms, and no running water, but I was blessed with good parents.

I attended a one-room school known as North Fork, then attended a one-room high school for two years known as Oldtown High School. It had one room and one teacher, just like four other one-room high schools in the county at that time. I went on to graduate from Greenup County High School in 1931. That high school was located twenty miles away, and there were no school buses because of road conditions. For my junior and senior years, a neighbor fixed up his cattle truck with seats and took us to Greenup High School.

My family borrowed fifty dollars from Greenup Bank to get me started to college. I worked my way through four years of college at Morehead State College, graduating in 1935. I was on my way, really thinking I could make a difference.

When I got a job as a one-room school teacher, my first school was Oldtown, and my next one-room school where I taught was Long Branch. My last teaching job in one-room schools was at Tunnel, where I taught for two years. I taught in Greenup County during the years 1934–54. During those years I also served as director of pupil personnel for ten years. When the new superintendent was chosen, I was fired, along with all office personnel. After that, beginning in 1954, I got a job just like the previous one, this time in the Russell Independent school system. I was there until 1976, when I retired.

All total I served in these school systems for forty-one years. Teaching school is a vital profession, and thankfully my four daughters followed in my steps.

Emma Walker, Eddyville

I was born August 26, 1925, in Hickman County, Tennessee. My father was William Cathey Baker, and my mother was Sarah Virginia Woody, who was from Obion County, Tennessee. I had five siblings—four brothers and one sister, and I'm the only survivor. All the schools I attended were larger than one-room. We lived in Centerville, Tennessee, for a period of time, but my first schooling was at Shady Grove, Hickman County. I rode on horseback behind one of my brothers, or when weather was cold or raining, we rode in a buggy. I sat on the floorboard at my brother's feet, wrapped in a quilt.

Mr. Eugene Glenn, superintendent of Lyon County Schools, called me and asked if I would consider teaching at Hebron to finish out that year, 1959. So my husband, Doyle, and I told the superintendent that I would. Doyle's great-grandfather gave the land on which the Hebron School was built. When it came school time the next year, Mr. Glenn asked me if I would teach again that year. So I signed a contract to teach that year, and at the end of that year the rural schools were consolidated. Of course, the students were bused into Eddyville then. So that was my beginning to kind of get my feet wet!

After teaching a short time, I was encouraged to go ahead and become a certified teacher. Early on I completed two years of college at Abilene Christian College, Abilene, Texas. I went to Murray State College and got my bachelor's degree, and was also teaching in Crittenden County at Frances Elementary at that time.

Superintendent Louis Leitchfield kept coming to the school, where I was teaching fifth grade, and was really happy as a fifth-grade teacher. Every time he came out there, he came to my room and talked to me about going into special education. He said, "We've got some students in the county that are considered special education students, but we don't have a certified teacher."

That was the beginning of special education programs anywhere, so I started as special education teacher in Crittenden County, and you might say the pioneer of all the programs that were started. I taught special education for twenty-four years, during which time I went ahead and got a master's degree, then became fully certified as a special education teacher.

If students have an excellent mentality and are motivated by parents, they can learn rapidly and be challenged to excel at their grade level or beyond. Younger students learn from the older ones and profit by seeing and hearing what they are doing, like reciting poems or in spelling bees and math competition. Many of these students have done well in the business world and diverse occupations, and others have been good providers for their family, are well respected, and have contributed much to society. It is such a reward to see these students in later life and learn of their successes, and then [they] give *me* credit for the impact I had on their lives.

Joyce Williams Ward, Campbellsville

I was born in Cumberland County, January 1938, and went to Howard's Bottom School in that county, 1944–52, from first through eighth grades. Subsequently I attended Cumberland County High School and graduated in 1956. After that I went to Western Kentucky University for one year; then the next year I went to Campbellsville College. I went to Campbellsville for two years, graduated in 1958, then taught one year in Cumberland County at Smiths Grove one-room school. When they made Campbellsville into a four-year college, I went back and graduated in 1962.

I got married, then taught first grade part-time at Greensburg Elementary School in 1959. They had an overflow of first graders. The next year I taught at Russell Creek School, Green County, then at Glenview School the next year.

I graduated from Western with a master's degree in 1968 and Rank 1 in 1971.

All total, I taught thirty-four years in Green County schools, one year in Cumberland County, and one year at Christian School in Taylor County. Twenty years of that time were spent teaching kindergarten in Green County.

Bige R. Warren, Barbourville

I was born December 26, 1937, on Roaring Fork of Stinking Creek, Walker, Kentucky, Knox County. There were thirteen family members, so we were a large family. Seven of us siblings are still living.

I attended Carnes Elementary School, a one-room school, then I graduated from Knox Central High School in 1958. I attended Cumberland College, Williamsburg, for one summer. I didn't have the money to go on to school, so I began teaching in a one-room school at Callebs Creek. They needed two teachers to fill two one-room schools, and I was one of them. My first year of teaching was in 1959–60 at Callebs Creek, a one-room school. My pay for that year was $137 each month. My next year of teaching was at Alex Creek, 1960–64, also one-room. I taught there for four years. After that I taught social studies at DeWitt Elementary here in Knox County. I also taught one year in Ohio.

I continued going to college, taking Saturday classes, night classes, and summer classes. During the next five years I achieved four years of college credit, and taught five years. I never went to college for a full year, but I finally got my B.S. degree in elementary education from Cumberland College, 1965.

I attended Eastern Kentucky University and received a master's degree, then enrolled at Union College to do my Rank 1 in principalship. I was never a principal, but after teaching for ten years, I started working for the state teachers organization, known as KEA. I worked for them for thirty-six years and retired about two years ago, 2006.

Betty Garner Williams, Campbellsville

I was born in 1932 in Cumberland County next to where the lake and park are now located. I went to a one-room school called Chestnut Grove for eight years, then graduated from high school in Burkesville in 1950. I enrolled in Campbellsville College, a two-year college, to get a degree that made me eligible to begin teaching. I graduated from there in 1952, then started teaching.

I taught at a one-room in Taylor County, located on Highway 70. The school was known as Farmers, and the building is still there. I soon got married to Russell Williams, and we lived in the western part of Kentucky for one year. I taught third grade at Pembroke, but it was not a country school. I gave my notice that I would be leaving before Christmas that year because we had bought a farm back in Taylor County.

We came back in early 1954 and moved to where we now live in Tebbs Bend on the Green River. During the next year, 1954–55, I taught at a school known as Meadow Creek, and that was the last year they had school there. There were only nine students in school there that year.

After our son, Greg, was born, and when consolidation was completed in 1956, I came back and began teaching as a first-grade teacher and remained there until 1991. I taught all those years except for a couple of years when Greg was little.

Marguerite Wilson, Leitchfield

I was born December 10, 1917, in Grancer, Butler County. My dad, Fieldon Woosley, was in World War I and was at Camp Taylor at that time. My mother, Beulah Embry, who left school to be married at age fifteen, was in Louisville at the time, but came back home in Butler County for my birth. I was born in the same house in which my mother and her mother were also born.

I went to Caneyville School during my elementary years. Our family moved there in 1921. That school was independent, thus not a part of the Grayson County system at that time. The school had grades 1 through 12, and I did all my schooling there. We had a superintendent then, as well as a principal, because we were not in the county system. The year I graduated from high school, it was still an independent school. I am so thankful I was valedictorian of my senior class that year in high school.

I always wanted to be a teacher, even from my early childhood. I went to Campbellsville College in 1935 and was there during two semesters and a summer term. After that I went to Western in Bowling Green where I received my provisional elementary certificate in 1937, after one semester and a summer term.

I taught at Goff's one-room school my first year, at Millwood, a two-room school, my second year, and my third year was at Walnut Grove, a one-room school. The Walnut Grove School was placed in the hands of a special organization, and the building is still standing in pretty good shape. Some schoolchildren are still taken there to see it and hear someone talk.

All total, I taught for twenty-eight years. I still get a retirement check, thank goodness!

A lot of my immediate family members taught schools across the years, and my youngest son became a doctor.

Mamie Wright, Tompkinsville

I was born August 13, 1915, to Tom and Effie Howard in northern Monroe County, and I still have the ring Daddy gave me that had my initials on the inside of the ring. He said, "I'll give you this if you will wear it." Well, I have worn it ever since he gave it to me. I would feel lost without it.

After finishing going to Hamilton one-room school, I went to Tompkinsville High School. We rented houses there in Tompkinsville and would take enough supplies from home to last a week. The rooms didn't cost much. After I graduated from high school in 1932, I went to college at Western but didn't obtain a degree at that time. I just taught and got what was called a life certificate, so I thought I'd be a teacher for life.

After that, even if you had your own life certificate, you'd have to go back and renew your degrees at different times to raise your salary. When I started teaching I was paid sixty-seven dollars each month.

Across the years I taught at Hamilton, Rock Bridge, Norman, Merryville, Oak Hill, Union Hill one-room schools, then ten years at Joe Harrison Carter Elementary. All total, I taught forty-two years.

Index of Stories by County